QUESTIONING CANCER

A brief insight into modern healthcare and the alternative treatments seldom granted

Questioning Cancer
By Giuliano D'alessandro

Published 2018 by Sazmick Books
Web: www.sazmickbooks.com

Author email: giulianod80@gmail.com

© Copyright 2018 Giuliano D'alessandro. All rights reserved.
No part of this book may be reproduced, stored in a retrieval system, or transmitted by any means without the written permission of the author.

Please note: The views in this book are not necessarily those of the publisher.

British Library Cataloguing-in Publication Data.
A catalogue record for this book is available from the British Library.

ISBN: 978-1-912400-09-6 (Paperback)
ISBN: 978-1-912400-10-2 (Ebook)

Printed and bound in the UK
using sustainable resources

Disclaimer: I feel the need to make readers aware that i have NO qualifications in the field of medicine and that the words expressed in this book should not be taken as medical advice. We should all be doing our own homework so that we may break free from intellectual laziness. Draw your own conclusions and please read up on additional material that has been written by educated professionals willing to challenge the status quo.

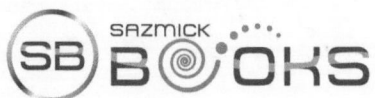

QUESTIONING CANCER

A brief insight into modern healthcare and the alternative treatments seldom granted

Giuliano D'alessandro

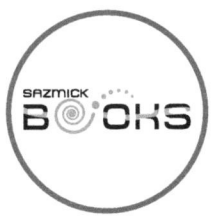

DEDICATION

For Sue

*"Your spirit is at peace now, and nature will guide and protect you,
for your next journey has only just begun.
May the pain that drifted away from your being
leave only love & truth, lighting your path back to the stars."*

DEDICATION

ACKNOWLEDGEMENTS

Thank you to Sazmick books, whose help and support has made this all possible...

And with thanks to those who care enough to question the norm and have the courage to do so; you know who you are.

CONTENTS

Dedication..v
Acknowledgements.....................................vii
Introduction..xi

Chapter 1: What We Eat.. 1
Chapter 2: Sugars.. 15
Chapter 3: The Power of Water.............................. 21
Chapter 4: The Milk Myth...................................... 35
Chapter 5: EMR/EMF Dangers................................ 41
Chapter 6: Vaccination: Fear, Myth, and Belief........... 55
Chapter 7: Herbs, the Lost Knowledge.................... 69
Chapter 8: Dis-ease.. 75
Chapter 9: The Incredible Healing Properties Of Cannabis.. 93
Chapter 10: Conclusion.. 105

Resources

Introduction

I felt compelled to write this book after witnessing an increasing number of family members, friends, and those in society all around us lose their lives to chronic illness. I became conscious of the passive acceptance of inefficient treatments within Western cultures specifically, and how we are led to believe that we receive the most comprehensive treatments for diseases possible. I started this journey out of curiosity and discovered how fellow humans from around the world had claimed to be healed from cancer, or at the least largely benefited, through alternative methods of medication. The curative statements and documented results in alternative disease treatment from those qualified in the field of medicine are staggering, and yet still controversial, in their conclusions. Unconventional treatment methods wrongly receive little coverage from the media as they can be unpopular with the status quo. With ever-growing numbers succumbing to cancer, the compiled evidence of long-term healing and side-effect free treatment protocols found within this book, and those found within the wider field of research available to us, can and do show how so many are not born out of false hopes. In the time I spent with friends and family going through orthodox cancer treatments, I was seeing people I cared about suffering, either physically, emotionally, or both. This made me want to find answers for them. In my quest to do so, I took to reading books and medical papers*[1], and it quickly became apparent to me that even our healthcare system is sick. The more questions I asked, the more I found, which led me to connect with people who had experiences and success of using alternative medicines. What became clear to me was that the modern and mainstream responses to cancer treatment were failing to include countless other forms of treatment that we could truly benefit from. I think it's important to note that I am not pointing the finger here at any particular consultant or practitioner of medicine but rather laying out an observation of what I consider to be failings of a broken system. Protective institutes, such as the FDA (food and drug administration), are in charge of guarding medicine for public consumption, yet simply cannot regulate effectively anymore, thus allowing corporations the privilege to set their own parameters.

Forgotten treatment methods have produced documented results that speak volumes to anyone wishing to listen and engage in critical thinking. Any medicine that challenges the norm is rarely granted a platform to present positive or consistent findings to a broader community, so that we may all be privy to the possibilities of this world. For many decades now, doctors have been managing the symptoms of disease whilst neglecting to understand the root

---

1   *(referenced in the index)*

issues which, in turn, has added to the growing number of cancers globally. We now live in an age where information has never been so easily accessible; it is literally at our fingertips now, while in almost any place, and at any time. We have access to a huge number of publications and chronological data that could, if acknowledged, allow further investigation into the alternative field of treatment and be made readily available for sufferers. The approaches described in this book are currently still well-documented and yet, at the same time, discouraged by the medical establishment as they do not fit the present program for medication in the modern world. Not only that, but these remedies will not cough up the billions of pounds needed to prop up what has become a vast empire for the manufacturing of pharmaceutical drugs. Are we becoming entrenched in corporate untruths believed to be true? The following pages of information merely challenge the existing acceptance of limited medical treatments that are not without harmful side-effects.

This book offers a way of looking at the world that you may not be used to, or perhaps you are unaware of, but don't worry, I was the same. Who is it that really benefits from modern mainstream treatments; the patient or the drug company? I wish to raise questionable doubt against chemotherapy, radiation, and surgery being the odd few answers we are provided when struck with illness. Valid solutions already exist and are simply not debated on an open platform for society to draw its own conclusions without being subject to prejudice, ridicule, greed, or prosecution. The clique in medicine conformity is ever more visible and has become its own religion, cutting down any who question its faithful believers. When a belief is entrusted without question or investigation, it is then possible to believe nothing else legitimate exists beyond that realm of perception, and you have been bamboozled. Thankfully, the human race has made it this far to the 21st century. This achievement has come from centuries of struggle; exposure to a host of climatic changes, geological shifts, the rise and fall of great civilisations and yet, this all happened without artificial drugs made by man. The argument here may be, "Well, we all live longer now thanks to modern medicine". Yet I also think we suffer longer, too. Although it is clear that millions of people have survived premature death from modern medical intervention relating to trauma, broken bones, and near fatal injury - this claim is not in dispute here - what is ultimately being questioned by this book are the restricted ways in which somebody can be healed. Surely all possibilities available to us in this tangible reality and all options to solve issues should be laid out on the table and identified honestly for each individual choice in what is a vibrant, resourceful, mysterious, and amazing world? This era of treatment exclusion is causing us a great injustice to our potential; we need to show honesty through moral duty in our actions and decisions if we are to truly move forward. If there is no benefit from alternative medicine, why do drug companies continue to replicate the blueprint found within nature? And why are so many people around the globe experiencing greatly enhanced results by turning away from mainstream treatments? Could we potentially save billions of pounds by simply harvesting that which already exists, using sustainable solutions for the future of the human race? Unconventional choices can consist of natural mediums little publicised that could be exploited for self-healing or professional administration, making it conceivable to increase your

Introduction

chances of triumph over illness beyond the limitations of orthodox medicine. I firmly believe we are currently being offered average treatments and that we should both be demanding more from our healthcare and learning for ourselves the abundance of solutions that nature has to offer. We can take responsibility for ourselves.

The material here can make it plausible to take back our personal power, become aware of the knowledge that will help us restore our unique relationship with the Earth, and uncover what continues to be ignored. I want to share what I have found so that you, the reader, may draw your own conclusions. By implementing changes to our perception, we can achieve amazing, yet simple, solutions, turning the impossible into possible.

Chapter 1
What We Eat

"Let food be thy medicine and thy medicine be thy food."
- Hippocrates

Organically grown food was the only way humans cultivated for thousands of years, and everything we used to digest - be it meat or plant - had no man-made chemicals added since agriculture was introduced.

20th century by-products, mostly from the petroleum industry, introduced pesticides to farmers to increase crop yield against pests and supply a steady demand for chemical resistance that set in motion the multi-billion pound synthetic fertiliser market we see today. The inherent problem with pesticides, herbicides, and fertilisers is that the more you use them to increase crop production and control pests, they, in turn, deplete natural minerals and vital nutrients within the soil. Crops become weaker, yet hungrier, over time for more chemical fertilisation and, in our unashamed use, we have created crop fertiliser addiction. Chemical man-made fertilisers are destroying the very source of natural energy and nourishment that plants take up in their root systems; glyphosate present in herbicides can block nutrient uptake so that a crop may not be able to absorb the optimum amount of nourishment from the minerals in the soil. It is worth noting that glyphosate marketed as "Roundup" is also found in shop-bought weed killer and has had a long history of dispute regarding its safety. Although concerns rage on globally, the EU Commission of Appeal has renewed its licence for a further five years despite a petition signed by 1.3million EU citizens calling for it to be banned. Over the course of the last 70 or so years, agricultural land has been exhausted from a measurable amount of life-giving nutrients that were available to us pre-20th century.

The increase of harmful chemicals used on the products we buy have turned the soil where our produce grows into an inferior growing medium, lacking optimum nutrients, vitamins, and laced with an increasing amount of hormone disruptors and carcinogens.

The organic movement came as early as the late 1940s in direct opposition to an increased use of pesticides and synthetic fertilisers. People already knew then that spraying our food would lead to health problems, and that was over half a century ago. Organic food has been growing in recognition in recent years and its impact on shopping trends has provided a sustainable industry for some and divided opinions for others.

"There is a growing shift in consumer purchasing towards organic food. Several studies have found that organic food contained more nutrients than conventional food, with higher levels of various minerals and vitamin C. These studies and similar have been conducted all over the world with results becoming self-evident about the benefits of organic over conventional. A large proportion of society is very unaware of the extras included when buying fruit, vegetables, and meat that has not been certified organic."[1]

The UK organic market is seeing strong growth in 2017 and is worth over £2 billion. Conscious consumers are helping to drive the figures of this market up, although what I find unreasonable is the legislation in place to produce under organic conditions, leading to a pricier end product for what should be a consistent standard across all food production. What upsets me is the division within society associated to organic living, as its higher price can exclude a large proportion of shoppers. Organic farmers pay a high price to adhere to strict regulations and they do not receive subsidies, unlike conventional farming practices. There is no incentive for farmers to become sustainable and we are funding damaging farming methods that cost us all more than we think. For every £1 spent on food by shoppers, another equal amount is quietly taken from us. A report on the hidden cost of UK food further states that the extra costs are not paid for by the food businesses that create them and are not even included within the retail price.

"Instead, they are passed on to society in a range of hidden ways

— meaning that UK consumers are, in effect, paying twice for their food." - The Hidden Cost of UK Food

I don't think the cost of organic is justified. What I mean by this is that if we incentivised sustainable practices, then we would all know we are receiving clean, chemical-free produce at affordable prices for all.

Intensively reared livestock are routinely fed antibiotics to stave off ill health; by a continuation of eating this type of meat, people can develop a reduced immunity from overexposure to antibiotics. Bacteria that become overexposed to synthetic antibiotics also become increasingly resistant to them.

The British Medical Association has stated that:

"The risk to human health of antibiotic resistance is one of the major health threats that could be faced in the 21st Century."

Through the use of synthetic chemicals, we are allowing and creating further resistance for bacteria that eventually ends up being labelled a super bug. What is the root cause of these new mutations and can they be prevented?

Eating organic is one way to safeguard your family's health, especially as we live in a world becoming ever more polluted and stained by unnatural chemicals. In our quest for innovation, we seem to have forgotten how important our diets are and to truly understand both the potential of certain foods and what effect they have on the human system. We should learn the remarkable effects that full nutrient rich diets can give us, including the ability to heal by strengthening the immune system alone. We expose ourselves daily to harmful chemical substances and toxins which are becoming increasingly difficult to escape from. Making small changes can, and do, make a difference. Organic food seems more costly to purchase and, yet, with conventional farming there are the hidden costs involved that are paid for by us eventually. Organic food can promote better animal husbandry and welfare than conventional farms, and leads to a greater understanding of how food affects humans and animals.

"The organic vs non-organic debate has rumbled on for decades now but the evidence from this study is overwhelming -organic food is higher in antioxidants and lower in toxic metals and pesticides."... "But this study should just be a starting point. We have shown without doubt there are composition differences between organic and conventional crops, now there is an urgent need to carry out well-controlled human dietary intervention and cohort studies, designed to identify and quantify the health impacts of switching to organic food." -Professor Carlo Leifert

The ongoing argument for organic and conventional foods always comes down to the benefit and whether it is really better for us. It's not until you commit to investigating the value of organic against conventional that the facts and moral obligation toward food products start to unravel. Every living species on Earth benefits from organic farming and that is why we should look at the wider picture of who benefits to include both animals and the environment, not just us. Conventional and mass produced foods and meat are resource-hungry and becoming ever more tainted with growth hormones, antibiotics, lower standards of animal husbandry, not to mention the growing subject of waste disposal. Organic produce is at the other end of the spectrum of food production where time, patience, commitment to care, and the use of strict regulation brings forth higher quality goods that as science is now confirming are richer in the viable nutrition that we need to sustain good health. The University of Newcastle committed to a study of organic vs non-organic using a systematic literature study, and their conclusions showed that organic crops have significantly higher antioxidant qualities - up to 60% over conventional - and lower toxic heavy metal content. The study published in The British Journal of Nutrition used an extensive analysis of 343 peer reviewed publications but, interestingly, the UK Food Standards Agency (FSA) stated in 2009, after commissioning a study based on only 46 publications, that there is no substantial difference or nutritional benefit from organic food.

Institutes such as the FSA are in place to protect the health and well-being of a nation, yet simply do not include enough data to draw accurate conclusions from and, more often than not, their policies favour big agribusinesses. Plants in their natural state were put on our planet to be used by us and all living things to promote life through nourishment and healing. Everything the body needs to thrive and repel illness comes from the earth itself and evidence clearly shows us that our diets reflect greatly whether we succeed in health or create breeding grounds for man-made degenerative diseases (diseases that we create ourselves).

When we ingest a plant or herb for healing reasons, we obtain the full display of compounds which gives plants their excellent healing qualities, thus leading to little or no side-effects in the correct doses, of course. Helping to make a conscious effort in support of our food industry in sustainable ways allows us to increase our knowledge of what we eat, and knowing exactly where it comes from can protect-our environment for future generations yet also improve our quality of life now, leading to fewer health problems and helping to prevent an increasing drain on our national health system. Herbs and plants have a tried-and-tested history, as their use has prevented mankind from extinction for thousands of years.

The true value of plant matter for health should not be underestimated by our 21st century minds, as understanding a plant-based diet healing safety record and efficacy against illness will definitely leave a competent mind questioning our mainstream reasoning and acceptance of modest treatments. The World Health Organisation estimates that 80% of humans can rely on herbal medicines for their primary health needs as, similarly, 70% of German physicians offer plant-based medicine to their patients. This choice is non-existent to sufferers in the UK. Why?

Over 100 of the prescription drugs available on the market today actually derive from plant origins, but the synthesis of natural products ultimately renders them unbalanced under natural law. The inadequacy of modern medicine is its often extreme side-effects that all too commonly create further complications and not a swift remedy.

I would like to see further independent and unbiased studies performed on organic and conventional farmed foods. The results, I believe, will only add weight to the benefits of organic but, until this time, there is still a known accumulative risk from eating food that has had chemicals added to its growing stage for only one sole purpose; to gain profit. This is important to understand. Farmers have been duped by large scale fertilisation techniques which ultimately benefits the companies involved while humanity's nutrition disappears. I really feel that, as a society, we need to question the motivation of chemical organisations to determine if the temporary solutions offered for profit's sake are actually viable for a sustainable future where our children's children may have the best nourishment to help them grow. As an even further consideration, perhaps another answer lies in vegetarianism whereby the rights of animals can be restored to the level that would eradicate all harm and death. We have been led to believe that meat in our diet is important, but what is clear is that, providing our vegetables are grown in organic conditions, and are rich in the vital nutrients the human body requires, then we could have more than enough to sustain life for all on Earth. Producing quality over quantity should be a primary goal, which is completely achievable.

There are many things we should learn about the daily consumption of various non-foods, medicines, and chemicals that have found their way into our daily lives. If we fail to question their use or benefit, how will we know if they are good for us or not?

The Modification of Foods

We are told by experts that genetically modified organisms (foods derived from organisms that are genetically altered and modified in a way that is not naturally occurring) will end starvation and are, above all, safe to consume. These statements, frequently used by GM promoters, are fantasies based upon improper studies which exclude negative results far too often to be anywhere close to transparent with their evidence on long-term effects for all life on Earth. The altering of genetic code so a company may patent its final product is the racket hidden within bioscience; a new problem is created within the food production industry, leading farmers to believe the solution is an engineered seed with heavy price tags and they often become contractually bound into an unsustainable loop. An engineered crop is designed to be resistant to specific herbicides and pesticides. The process starts by buying seeds which you are not allowed to store and save each year, and the seed pushers then sell you the chemicals to spray upon your crops which are resistant to the ingredients of the patented chemicals. Clever science or good business? Farmers are becoming increasingly dependent on big business, which is sending the agricultural industry spiralling into an exceptionally unsustainable process. Once locked into contract with companies such as Monsanto, who have been at the forefront of biotechnology and food modification since their founding 116 years ago, there seems like no way out. Age-old and sustainable agricultural practices are being forced out from human knowledge, including the contamination of natural biodiversity. The case of "David versus Goliath" - a documentary about Percy Schmeiser - brings the true reality of companies like Monsanto to life. A common scenario faced by U.S and Canadian farmers are mafia-like tactics backed by giants of industry willing to crush any competition for profit domination. The very leaders of the biotech enterprise and fellow campaigner institutes or government bodies are reading a script crafted and produced by business for business which sells us an alleged sustainable solution yet creates the exact opposite. We have no more need for GMO than we do nuclear weapons; they both cause levels of destruction in different ways and are yet equally cataclysmic.

As a consumer, I had no idea about the negative health impacts associated with GM food; for instance, the same companies selling us the GM lie are the same companies that sold us DDT, Agent Orange, and promoted just how safe PCBs were. In my opinion, Monsanto, Bayer, Syngenta, Du Pont, and Dow have all sold us lies about alleged beneficial gains from GM products and chemical production with little debate or even correct regulation regarding the impacts of modifying life. The introduction of genetic modification within agriculture is not dissimilar to releasing a contaminate upon nature.

The perception that GM can save us is giving the green light to biotech companies that are polluting nature with new organisms and thus changing the equilibrium that flora and fauna have survived with until now. In fact, genetic manipulation has been shown to alter DNA code and produce highly questionable negative side-effects in animal studies.

The art of working with nature which has prevented our demise for millennia is being lost to the people and, ultimately, minimising choices for both farmers and end consumers. We are being sold the fake science of Frankenfoods so that a few companies may dominate the food market.

There is enough food production on Earth to feed at least 10 billion people. The problem is not in volume production but in the way wealthy countries distribute, and how modern societies waste millions of tons of food each year through unconscious consumption which, in turn, creates food markets that are not affordable and accessible to those who languish in poverty whilst observing the inequality outcome of a capitalist gorging system within our societies.

In 1998, a lawsuit forced over 40,000 secret FDA memos into the public domain for scrutiny, and what became clear was that the FDA had been lying regarding the safety of genetic modification. The claims that GM was safe to consume conflicted greatly with the internal staff findings who were in charge of regulatory responsibility, as not only was genetic modification deemed unsafe, but it was also found that their use could lead to allergies, increased toxins, new diseases, and depleted nutrient uptake.

These internal findings were raised with FDA superiors with the suggestion that long-term studies were needed to clarify any negative health outcomes, yet were ignored. What is appalling within so many alleged regulation agencies is the dire situation of conflicts in interest which overturn safety in favour of power and profit. At the time of these findings, Michael Taylor was in charge of policies at the FDA and also happened to be Monsanto's former lawyer and vice president.

The illusion of regulation from the FDA was all that was needed for the biotech industry to continue its domination, when in fact there was no regulation imposed whatsoever. The free reign for industry and its commitment to profit, not safety, is a clear sign that protection agencies have lost the capacity to regulate in a concise and proper manner. Corporations are the ones wielding the power to influence illusions of safety which are accepted as scientific fact, not the pursuit of truth.

Labelling of GMO products in the UK is currently mandatory, which allows us the choice to avoid certain products if we wish. One of our powers as consumers is conscious consumerism, and to make ourselves aware of what exactly we are getting for our money. However, what is interesting is that out of the top 10 UK supermarkets, only one is fully committed to sourcing GM-free meats and dairy across its range. It's a shame that access to such untainted food comes at a recognisable cost which unfortunately falls outside the spending powers of the general population. The inclusion of whether an animal has been fed a GM diet on product labelling should be mandated and yet this still remains to be seen. We know that feeding animals a GM diet has led to serious side-effects within farmed animals, and studies performed on rodents shows that third generation offspring are completely infertile. Thus, independent testing gives us the evidence needed to, at the very least, ask some serious questions about GMO safety to both the manufacturers and the agencies that are allegedly protecting us from harm.

Chapter 2
Sugars

Refined processed sugar is possibly one of the most dangerous foods any human can put into their body which has become evident in child obesity rates and tooth decay statistics. White or brown processed sugar has no nutritional value whatsoever, is devoid of vitamins and minerals, and consists of only empty calories.

Sugar in its natural state comes from raw cane or sugar beet. Raw sugar has to undergo a vigorous process by which all of its health promoting benefits is put through extensive heat treatments that kills any goodness that once existed. The liquid from washed and shredded cane stalks is boiled and treated with chemicals to remove impurities.

It is then moved to large tanks to evaporate water content and put in a centrifuge machine to form the thick syrup into crystals. The crystals are then transported to a sugar refinery where it is boiled and, yet again, more chemicals are added. It then continues its journey through a filtration process using bone char, which is made from cow or pig bones, and on to its final stage where it is centrifuged again, thereby producing the end result which is refined white sugar. Brown sugar is created by adding molasses before putting it in the centrifuge. This whole process has practically annihilated all life out of its original state, leaving the final product useless for consumption. Digesting these types of sugars has a whole host of detrimental effects on the body; it causes a mineral imbalance and contributes to migraines, mental disorders, depression, diabetes, arthritis, and disease. It creates an acidic environment within the body which, in turn, depletes essential nutrients and vitamins that are imperative for a fully-functioning immune system that helps us ward off colds and flu. To metabolise refined sugar, the chemical process steals calcium from bones and teeth, leading to tooth decay and osteoporosis. It has negative effects on behaviour, linking its overconsumption to violent behaviour, hypertension, and learning impediments, along with obesity and allergies amongst children.

Sugar is also highly addictive, much along the same lines as some narcotics with very similar withdrawal symptoms. Refined sugar is essentially a worthless non-food that has dire consequences for the human system; it has all the hallmarks of a poison and can be lessened from a daily need to sweeten. Natural sweeteners are available; honey, Rapadura, Xylitol, rice malt, and barley malt are tasty alternatives.

Rapadura is a South American sugar that is extracted using a press and heated at very low temperatures, and this way of extraction retains minerals and nutrients. It is organically produced with no added chemicals. Rapadura has approximately 28g/kg mineral salts, whereas refined white sugar has approximately 300mg/kg. This is a very good sugar with a caramel taste, is organically produced, and is relatively cheap to buy. Organic cane sugar retains some beneficial minerals, and switching to alternatives instead of processed sugar will contribute to a sustainable future. It's difficult to know what's available to us outside of mass market products unless we become consciously aware consumers.

Aspartame is a synthetic sweetener found in a wide variety of dry foods and drink. It was created by accident in 1965 while a chemist working for the company Searle was testing an anti-ulcer drug. Neuroscience researcher Dr John W. Olney and Consumer Attorney James Turner filed objections against its use in 1974, so its widespread use was put on hold. That was until Monsanto took over the business reigns in 1985, by which time legislation was hurried along by a Mr Donald Rumsfeld, who helped to approve usage for both food and beverages.

Many reactions to aspartame are serious; there are up to 90 documented different associated symptoms being caused by this chemical poison ranging through dizziness, nausea, numbness, weight gain, rashes, depression, insomnia, vision problems, hearing loss, vertigo, memory loss, and joint pain. Researchers and physicians studying the adverse effects of aspartame have stated the following chronic illnesses can trigger or worsen, too; Chronic Fatigue Syndrome, Parkinson's disease, Alzheimer's, brain tumours, Multiple Sclerosis, epilepsy, mental retardation, lymphoma, and even birth defects. Aspartame is made up of aspartic acid, phenylalanine, and methanol, all of which combine to make an excitotoxin, a chemical which excites neural cells to death. Aspartame affects brain function, causes damage to cells, and is known to be carcinogenic, so can pave the way for cancer.

A 2013 re-evaluation by the European Food Safety Authority still categorised aspartame as safe, but their conclusions are a stark contrast to the many independent studies which affirm otherwise.

A known aspartame manufacturer, Monsanto was one of nine wartime producers of Agent Orange back in the Vietnam War. The long-term environmental and health effects were downplayed, which led military troops to pay the ultimate price. Most surprising about its use during the war was the unaccountability for damage claims where the U.S court system stated contractors of the chemical were not responsible. So who is?

Aspartame is now found in most fizzy pop, fruit juice drinks for children, diet yoghurt, and sweets, along with NutraSweet, VitaSweet, and Canderel sweeteners.

All metabolites of aspartame (formaldehyde, methanol, diketopiperazine, and formic acid) are toxic to the human body, and are especially toxic to the brain even in low consistent concentrations.

Needless to say, avoiding these toxic chemicals should become a priority, especially if you are suffering from an illness.

Aspartame really is a dangerous additive that is found in so many beverages and, to avoid it, you have to become chemically aware of what you are consuming. Conscious consumerism is our greatest power in avoiding harmful chemicals. There is enough evidence available to have aspartame removed from human consumption. Its continual use in the food and drink market is a disease catalyst and shows disregard from not only agencies that are supposed to be protecting citizens' health and regulating chemicals properly, but also industry for using cheap and toxic ingredients in the first instance. It is hard to determine what foods have aspartame in at first, but with keen reading of labels, you can avoid this offensive chemical and many others you may feel that are of no benefit to your well-being.

Chapter 3

The Power of Water

Water is one of the most underrated subjects regarding the well-being of human health. Chronic dehydration is an increasing problem that is responsible for many common symptoms, but the quality of water we drink is also very important.

Dehydration is a very common source of illness; it is said the average adult should be drinking 1–2 litres of good quality water every day, and more if you are unwell. This volume of water intake is under much scrutiny and seems to be a figure dreamt up by the bottled water industry. Even so, water is the second most vital life source you need after oxygen. Although the body is 70% water and the brain is 90% salt water, your body does not produce water or mineral salts and is forever losing these through respiration, perspiration, and urination daily. When you factor our modern diets into the equation, along with pollution, working in climate-controlled offices, and centrally-heated houses, 1-2 litres of water a day to help wash your system out seems like a more sensible idea than a necessity.

A daily regime of tea and coffee can dehydrate the body slightly as caffeine is a diuretic, making the body urinate more than usual and leading to a loss of fluids. How much caffeine can dehydrate is still a well-debated topic but, nevertheless, if you are trying to get well from illness, it is best to avoid all fluids and foods that may add any imbalance to your body, especially drinks containing caffeine which is a drug stimulant and of no benefit to a healing body. The Institute of Medicine has stated that caffeinated beverages can contribute to your daily water needs but it is my opinion that perhaps this conclusion favours the annual profits of the caffeinated industry far better than the health of a nation's people.

Our bodies need constant replenishment of water in order to enable chemical and electrical responses to deal with our day-to-day functioning quickly. If we don't keep the body topped up with clean water regularly, we effectively open a door to allow aches, disease, and illness to strike. If, like many Westernised humans, you do not eat enough fruit and vegetables, then cleaning your body's insides with regular water is common sense for diets in the West. Some symptoms of dehydration include aches and pains, high blood pressure and high cholesterol, constipation, headaches, dizziness, and loss of strength and stamina.

Water in our diets in a modern society has the ability to drastically reduce illness and help aid any healing process. The lack of recognition for the intake of a liquid so vital to our existence is like disregarding the need to breathe.

I mention the term "good water"; the wet stuff that comes out of our taps may look clean, the water companies will attest to the minimum requirements for safety and quality, and of course it is safe to drink, yet is it the best process we can offer for humanity? It certainly pays to add a home filtration unit to improve overall taste and to remove as much unwanted contaminates as possible. Putting a filtered glass of tap water next to tap water really does make you notice not only the smell of chlorine in ordinary tap water, but the improved taste of water that has been filtered. Why drink with chlorine?

Chlorine added to water supplies is a cheap solution, and that is all it is. It is effective and yet highly reactive with other substances which can form toxic compounds, including carcinogenic by-products. Although originally used as a weapon in World War I, its use today is considered normal for human consumption. We are slowly poisoning our bodies by the long-term consumption of chlorinated water, even though other viable yet more expensive solutions exist, such as ozone and colloidal silver that simply do not have the negative effects of bleaching. There really is no reason to chlorinate water supplies, yet we are stuck with the cheap non-solutions that public water services can get away with. Bottled water, over the course of a year, can make a dent in your wallet unnecessarily. In addition to not being particularly good for the environment by creating plastic bottles, the leaching of the chemicals used in creating plastics is a concern, especially when containers get warm in the sun. Bisphenol A (BPA) - a chemical used in the production of plastic bottles, amongst other products - has had a lot of press recently, as it is a synthetic oestrogen and a known endocrine disrupter. Avoiding this chemical is becoming a growing consensus but what of the other chemicals used in manufacturing plastics? The use of plastics on Earth is an increasing problem for the sustainability of all life on our planet, with its use affecting everything within the ecosystem regardless of its limited potential for recycling. Glass bottles do not leach and remain inert vessels that affect little, if any, of the stored liquid. Glass is far better for the environment than plastic and its high recycle rate should be much favoured by commerce for a balanced pollution-free environment.

Distilling water is an excellent method for removing the vast majority of impurities. For any water, distillation provides an equal level as, if not greater than, reverse osmosis. There are many arguments regarding the benefits of distilled water and all the negatives that persist seem to come from marketing battles within the water industry itself. In the published material on water distillation, it is apparent that distilled water is as pure as you could want to get domestic tap water. Although distillation removes all minerals and has a slightly acidic pH value, its use should not be disregarded, and I am aware of many people who celebrate its benefits. A long-held argument for anti-distillers is that distilled water has no mineral benefit and is considered empty water but, to this, the only reply would surely be that my minerals and nutrients come from fresh fruit and vegetables, not water alone. Adding a small amount of pink

Himalayan salt to your finished product will re-introduce over 75 trace minerals. Reverse osmosis is the reversal of the natural flow of osmosis. In a water purification system, the goal is not to dilute the salt solution, but to separate the pure water from the salt and other contaminants. When the natural osmotic flow is reversed, water from the salt solution is forced through the membrane in the opposite direction by application of pressure, thus the term 'reverse osmosis'. Through this process, we are able to produce pure water by screening out the salts and other contaminants. This method does waste water, but many still use RO as a pure water supply for their needs. If you are keen to change what you drink, then the cost of drinking good quality water does not have to be an expensive adventure. Another affordable way to avoid ingesting most of the pollutants is by using a simple charcoal water filtration unit for your tap water. An under-sink plumbed water filter for your cold water feed is effective at removing most harmful organisms; they are available with installation instructions and are simple to install for the average person with a toolbox. This inexpensive system will produce better quality drinking water for you and your family, but will still struggle at reducing excessive parts per million. Ideally, you need to look for filter sizes of 1 micron and below. Unless you have tried filtered water, you really don't know what you're missing out on taste-wise and for your health. Cheap supermarket water jug filters have expensive filter costs and do not remove enough of the heavy metals and harmful organisms due to having poor large-sized filters which still allow most metals and bacteria to pass through. These devices are a fad. Although you can see a visible residue left behind when using these types of filtration units, it is not nearly enough removal of wastes to provide you with a good cost-effective product. Avoid these filter jugs, as they are useless and rely on marketing far greater than processing quality H2O. Drinking clean water and clear water are totally different things, as what is happening inside the water is not apparent to the naked eye, but we can still taste and smell any differences with relative ease. Unfortunately, the vast majority of us believe that if you don't drop down dead instantly from ingesting something that may be harmful long-term, then, well... it must be safe to drink. Nearly all dietary choices are cumulative and affect us long-term. Each choice we make along our paths will shape the future that has not reached us yet. Alas, other devices use ceramic filters that remove most impurities. The main benefit of such a filter is that it works using gravity, meaning no power consumption and no waste water. It also alkalises the water, which is an added benefit for health. The British Berkefeld gravity water filter is well-known and uses ceramic filters as well, and the black filters available have a lifespan of over 22,000 litres which, in a small home, should easily last 10 years plus. They are incredibly easy to use and are one of the only filter companies to issue an international reduction scale of impurities to 99.99%. There is a vast choice of expensive machines available that claim remarkable results, but be cautious and do your research about everything you read including what you read here, as these ways written are not the only ways. There are alkaline and ionising machines which help reduce acidity within the body, increase oxygen intake, and can correct the body to a more alkaline environment, costing anywhere from £200 to £2000. Please be aware of what you are purchasing and be knowledgeable about your product, ask yourself what method will suit you best for pocket in the long-term, what it is you are wishing to remove from municipal water supplies, and how a filtered medium will be of use.

Fluoride Use

Fluoride, commonly referred to as sodium fluoride, is allowed to be put in our water supply and is a non-organic compound coming mainly from fertiliser and aluminium production waste, which is a processed industry by-product. This is not to be confused with naturally occurring calcium-fluorophosphate found in many foods. Calcium-fluorophosphate is easily assimilated by the body causing no harm, and is derived from wholefoods as an edible organic salt. Hydrofluorosilicic Acid, which is the waste product from the Phosphate industry, is being encouraged to be dumped in British water supplies as a convenient, cheap solution of disposal under the pretence of protecting dental decay. Unfortunately for us, it becomes retained within the body, leading to lower birth rates, sperm count, and testosterone levels, along with neurological problems such as Alzheimer's, Dementia, ADD, and a possible reduced IQ in children, as a recent study in China concluded. It affects the thyroid gland which causes disruption in the uptake of crucial iodine. There are many papers and a whole collection of scientific studies in favour of fluoridating water supplies, but this activity contradicts human rights issues and the sheer conduct of what is essentially mass medication is a violation upon a nation's water supply. The continued rhetoric surrounding the beneficial use of fluoride that comes from the FDA, FSA, DOH, and dentistry industry at large is a fraud; another popular accepted untruth that is feverishly peddled and defended by those that believe in it. This man-made chemical serves no purpose even existing and we should not ignore any government's decision to mass medicate a populace, considering the plethora of data that suggests not only is fluoride harmful long-term even in small quantities, but it is also morally wrong to overtly medicate those which do not need medicating using a chemical that is not an essential nutrient. We are told it is primarily used in the drinking supply as it is proven to prevent tooth decay, and this fabrication has become so ingrained in many a professions training that its defence is worrying and irresponsible. The actual benefits for its widespread use are remarkably minimal in comparison to the negative effects reported.

"Fluoride science is corporate science. Fluoride science is DDT science. It's asbestos science. It's tobacco science. It's a racket." Learn how The Mellon Institute, on behalf of Alcoa Aluminium, helped "prove" the safety of fluoride, just as they had with asbestos, by manufacturing fraudulent science for more than half a century in an effort to stem massive litigation against industry polluters."
-Christopher Bryson, Author of "The Fluoride Deception"

All of the various government-funded organisations who are certain they have our best interests at heart continue to ignore data proving otherwise; our bodies do not need waste material, and this action from authority is nothing short of an abuse against both our human rights and civil liberties. We are told by doctors and dentists alike that fluoride is a safe compound which has the ability to decrease dental decay, hence the reason for using it in toothpaste. It is found in nature where concentrations are less than 0.2ppm in the planet's fresh water systems, yet councils of men have given permission to dump up to 1.2ppm in some drinking supplies. Various studies have been conducted that prove the very opposite to the said benefits of fluoride, and conclusions have been, and are being, drawn showing there is no apparent proven results in reducing dental decay when using fluoride toothpastes often containing levels exceeding 1500ppm. Another side-effect of fluoride consumption is a problem known as dental fluorosis. Your teeth can form unattractive stains which are caused by the disturbance of enamel from excessive exposure to fluoride. Severe cases cause darkened areas on teeth which become rough and hard to clean. The government admit dental fluorosis is caused by fluoride, so do we really need this toxic substance put into our water supply? Fluoride is also used as a highly-effective rat poison in some European countries, offering instant extermination of rats with no antidote! Well, it must be good for us humans, then. There are fluoride-free toothpastes available to us that I have found more effective than the normal hyped-up over-marketed commercial junk or, better still, make your own toothpaste; there are many tutorials online. A UK law passed in 2003 allows health authorities to order private water companies to fluoridate the water supply. At present, about 5.5 million people drink fluorinated water, mainly in the North of the UK. Food can also be tainted with fluoride contained within the pesticide cryolite, which is used extensively in the US whereby the humble grape is a major fruit of contamination as it has received excessive spraying of this incredibly sticky substance. We should recognise that mass medication through municipal supplies is based on fabricated data and that the fertiliser industry is tainting our food with toxic chemicals, which is why organic foods can play an important role in healing the body from heavy metals and toxic overload. It is clear that if you want to be smart and ahead of the herders, you need to do something about it yourself and help protect your family's health. 97% of Europe has rejected water fluoridation, but why? The statements of rejection to fluoridate water supplies from 12 European countries need to be fully considered so that we may eradicate the heinous activity of dumping waste material into public water supplies.

"In point of fact, fluoride causes more human Cancer death, and causes it faster than any other chemical." -Dr Dean Burk PHD

Taking Filtration One Step Further

Viktor Schauberger, born in 1885, became a highly knowledgeable figure in the study of living water. He first pioneered what we now recognise as quantum, or subtle, energy changes and how they affect water. His ethos on life and how to work sustainably was to "observe nature and copy". He was a brilliant engineer and used his skills to create eco-friendly technology and energy devices that would help us refrain from using fossil fuels. He had a great understanding of nature and recognised water as a living energy for all life. He witnessed how, when water flows in rivers and over waterfalls, it follows the path of least resistance. He noted natural water courses are shaped by winding curves and shaded banks which helps protect it from direct sunlight, and its low temperature and natural flow helping preserve and support its energy. He perceived water to be the life blood of Earth, and his discoveries led him to design and construct devices which restore the energy into drinking water using a vortex system. He found two forms of motion in nature: outward, expanding flow that is used to break down, and inward-spiralling which nature uses to build up and energise. Using a simple vortex device, he was able to replicate nature's way of restoring energy to deficient water. Even when water is filtered using carbon and charcoal filtration units, the memory of the impurities removed remains in the water on a molecular level. The process of water distribution and extracting from reservoirs to a water company's treatment processes exposes water to a host of detrimental chemicals and pollutants. This interaction, which consists of electromagnetically charged information, becomes a murderous culprit to water molecules, rendering them lifeless of positively charged frequencies and the balanced information of energy so that it may give life. There is very little science dedicating time to this area of thinking which is restricting our view and how we believe that physical matter should be our concerns alone. Nature did not intend water to be forced through old pipes, picking up a host of containments, leaving scientifically measurable memory of all these previous forces upon it. There are a few vortex devices on the market, mainly by researchers who have carried on the work of Viktor Schauberger, which all are at varying prices but essentially have the same principle. The use of egg-shaped vessels has been around for millennia, and the ancients knew that storing in this way would keep liquids fresh and pure. Without any acknowledgement of what is found in UK tap water, it is inevitable that health issues continue to arise. Remember, every living thing on our planet needs energy rich water to survive and thrive. The quality of the water we drink in an ever-increasing polluted environment will become paramount to the safety and protection of our immune systems both now and in the future. It is a necessity for us all to become more aware of what we ingest on a daily basis and how this can directly affect our ability to function at our given optimum. We base our efficiency on reasonable clarity and bacterial reduction when we could be, in addition, offering fully-energised water that the body can easily assimilate. I understand that the not-too-distant future will present an environment where fresh water will become a highly prised commodity, as there is already evidence that governments and organisations are trading in water monopolies, including the theft of land to control its flow to the people at a very high price indeed.

Colloidal Silver

"Silver in various forms has been used in healing for centuries. The ancient Greeks and Romans used silver jars to keep stored liquids fresh. They wore silver frequently, perceiving that it maintained health. European royal families did not become as infected by the plague because they used silver utensils and ate off silver plates. And during the 1800s, American pioneers kept silver dollars in their milk jugs to prevent the milk from fermenting or spoiling. Silver coins were also dropped into water barrels to impede the growth of microorganisms and algae. One of the first recorded medical uses of silver dates back to 1834, when a German obstetrician named

F. Crede administered a 1% silver nitrate solution into the eyes of newborns to prevent blindness caused by eye infections. This practice continues today in hospitals around the world." [2]

Colloidal silver is a product that I have been using for over 5 years now, and it has proven its worth time and time again. Remember, there is no cure for the common cold but it can be prevented and lessened by what we eat and the steps we take to halt symptoms in their tracks. Another example is that of my daughter when she was unwell at 3 years old; she became quite exhausted and her body developed a nasty stye on each eye. We took her to a doctor for diagnosis confirmation and they gave us an eye spray which we were told would take almost 10 days to clear it up because of resistance to such current treatment these days. I knew there was a better more efficient way, so we used instead non-toxic, non-stinging 10ppm colloidal silver drops in each eye 3 times a day. Both styes were gone within 48 hours…

I also use it on cuts, burns, grazes, and for cleaning. As mentioned above, there is a wealth of uses for this amazing antibiotic/trace mineral.

There have been many case studies on its benefits at various universities and a whole lot more testimonials regarding its use on cancer patients and sufferers of HIV. Colloidal silver is safe to use for all ages, providing it is in low concentrations of no more than 12ppm for internal consumption. If you are suffering from a degenerative disease, you can use silver as you would a synthetic antibiotic, and it will help to protect your immune system safely along with the use of probiotics whilst not affecting the natural equilibrium your body undertakes when an attack from disease upon it is made. Silver generators are available online at very practical prices.

Buying it ready-made online is easy and the quality is very good from a UK supplier, which you can test yourself with the correct equipment, but ensure that you buy from a reliable source. Out of everything mentioned in this booklet, colloidal silver is the one product every household can benefit from; not only to help with family health but by assisting our environment if you use it instead of harsh cleaning chemicals which, as spoken about in a previous chapter, will eventually find their way into our water system.

"All truth passes through three stages. First, it is ridiculed. Second, it is violently opposed. Third, it is accepted as being self-evident." - Arthur Schopenhauer,

Chapter 4
The Milk Myth

For many years, I was under the impression that cow's milk was a good source of calcium for a human and generally a healthy staple drink full of good proteins that can be enjoyed in so many ways. I remember how my mum told me, and still hear mums today tell their children, to drink milk because it's good for them and will make their bones strong.

This illusion has been adopted by society for so long now in the belief that cow's milk is full of calcium, which strengthens our bones. This adopted belief came from the wonderful marketing tactics of the commercialised dairy industry. I wonder why, then, the US and UK, who consume regular amounts of cow milk and dairy products, have the highest rates of osteoporosis? Now, compare this to countries who consume very little dairy in their diets; they have exceptional bone density, far fewer cases of osteoporosis, and lower fracture incidents. The only processed milk available to society has been pasteurised, and this process can diminish the availability of calcium as well as destroying the enzymes needed to break down the milk in your body. Cows get their calcium from eating grasses to make their bones large, and the grass in turn has a high magnesium content that is crucial for the absorption of calcium. We drink cow's milk without the high magnesium content, which has already been absorbed by the cow. This prevents our bodies correctly assimilating the calcium that may be present. Essentially, you need a high magnesium content to absorb calcium - certainly in the amounts which are claimed by the current health authority. The dairy industry has been quick to capitalise on the fear of osteoporosis and bone fractures that affect a large proportion of the older society.

Mass dairy farming overtook the local farms and squeezed out small scale dairy producers to cope with the increased demand from supermarkets. This gargantuan task for sucking dry hormonal dairy cows became achievable through the use of high-processing rate machinery which, when introduced into the farming industry, changed the dairy farm forever. Raw natural milk has been consumed for centuries by humans around the globe; in this natural state, the enzymes needed to help humans digest milk are present along with the full bio available rich proteins that our bodies can utilise. Cow's milk, the liquid meat, should be treated with caution in all its becoming; the proteins present may actually leach calcium from the bones. When industry started imposing regulation on dairy products, pasteurisation was introduced, and this process kills the enzymes needed for us to digest milk efficiently. Pasteurisation does not kill all bacteria or sterilise the milk. Interestingly, cow's milk is allowed to have faeces in it, which, in itself, is a major source of bacteria. Milk is normally only pasteurised for 15 seconds at approximately 72 degrees Celsius. When you consider that sanitising water takes several minutes at 100 degrees Celsius, there certainly seems to be a huge disparity.

The EU currently allows 400,000,000 pus cells per litre of processed milk! It really is no wonder how milk turns sour so quickly and, in fact, doubles in bacteria every 20 minutes when left at room temperature.

"It's not natural for humans to drink cow's milk. Human milk is for humans. Cow's milk is for calves. You have no more need of cow's milk than you do rat's milk, horse's milk or elephant's milk. Cow's milk is a high fat fluid exquisitely designed to turn a 65 lb baby calf into a 400 lb cow. That's what cow's milk is for!" -Dr Michael Klaper MD

The statement above - when looked at logically - makes complete sense. We are humans, not calves. The battle with overcoming milk intake is, for some, the undeniably delightful taste to so many around the globe. Milk is a versatile substrate that we have all grown up with and remains familiar way into adulthood. The milk for each animal present on Earth is specifically formulated for the young of each individual species, dependant on their very unique requirements and necessities in reaching their prime.

Dairy is a highly-processed industry these days, processing large quantities of beef, milk, cheese and cream. The number of cows needed to produce such vast amounts of edible liquid meat is alarming; America alone has over 9 million dairy cows, and the UK has roughly 2.3 million. Intensive farming methods produce staggering amounts of animal waste (slurry) with millions of tonnes polluting rivers, streams, and lakes, not even mentioning the methane gas emitted by farmed animals, of which there are now 70 billion in factory farming. Beef still remains a massive contributor to our global pollution achievements that is, and has been, polluting our environment and bodies since mass production was introduced. Over 80 million tons of animal waste is produced in the UK alone every year, meaning farmers having to find a way to get rid of it instead of nature's way of recycling out in a meadow.

"There is compelling evidence, now published in top scientific journals and some of which is decades old, showing that cows' milk is associated, possibly even causally, with a wide variety of serious human ailments including various cancers, cardiovascular diseases, diabetes and an array of allergy-related diseases. And, this food contains no nutrients that cannot be better obtained from other far more nutritious and tasty foods." - Dr. Colin Campbell

Over 80% of milk is actually water, so this makes milk a very expensive white water. Casein, which forms over 75% of the protein in milk, is a strong binder that is used as a polymer to make plastics. It is also used to make glue, paints, and is present in thousands of processed foods as a binder. Casein is also a potent allergen that creates lots of mucus. Perhaps eating dairy is a strong promoter for the long list of allergies children face today? Most products containing dairy state milk as an allergen in bold on their product labelling within the UK; industry protects itself by actually acknowledging this fact, but it's up to us to realise this. It is hard to believe that such a staple part of our diet can cause damage to our bodies, but the impact dairy has on us is becoming increasingly noticeable to those in science along with nutritional awareness and, as more information is researched, the more action we can take to alleviate such problems arising from dairy consumption, not forgetting some of the horrendous conditions our bovine inmates have to suffer as a result of our collective unconsciousness. It is important to note that there are more humans in the world intolerant to the lactose in cow milk than not, so this should in itself speak volumes of how most human bodies reject the milk of another beast, especially one so eagerly exploited in the West. We do not have the same specific needs as a baby calf, so our bodies can react to lactose as an allergen which can, and in many cases, form the backbone of underlying health issues. Obesity is an increasing phenomenon, particularly in countries that consume a lot of dairy. Many other conditions can arise from dairy diets, for example, Mycobacterium paratuberculosis causes a bovine disease that cannot be killed by pasteurisation. The bacteria become cultured in the milk and can be passed onto humans.

In an article published by the Department for Environment, Food and Rural Affairs on 30 November 2009, they state:

"There is no statutory action taken, even in Northern Ireland where

the disease is notifiable, therefore any action taken is up to the owner. There is no effective treatment for Johne's Disease. Cattle that exhibit clinical signs are likely to be excreting large numbers of organisms capable of infecting other animals, especially calves in the herd."

So, how many of these organisms are not killed during the limited pasteurisation techniques employed by the dairy industry?

Startling information produced by the National Dairy Farm Magazine back in February 2002 proclaimed that 89% of dairy herds in the USA were infected with the leukaemia virus. Although government-funded studies affirm the UK free of bovine leukaemia, I would still regard the dairy industry, and even its weak processing efficacy, highly questionable.

Whatever the conflict of opinion in science and nutrition on dairy products are, it may be wise to be cautious of the dairy industry and decide for yourself whether there is any benefit of consuming cow's milk, perhaps considering an alternative if you have any ailments that dairy could be causing hindrance. If milk should remain in your diet, then organic milk should be explored. A UK study led by Newcastle University regarding organic milk vs conventional discovered that organic milk and meat contains more omega-3 by over 40% in comparison to conventional. A review of 196 papers found clear differences between the two. Try reducing your dairy consumption, as changing your diet can have huge impacts on your health.

Chapter 5
EMF/EMR Health Dangers

EMF stands for electromagnetic field and EMR for electromagnetic radiation. These forms of energy are invisible to the human eye and are silent to our ears, yet we know they are there. The physical fields of electrically-charged objects are becoming prolific within human activity, and questions need to be raised regarding their safety towards all life on Earth. The human body is electromagnetic which produces its own field, and this biological electrical capability enables information to travel to all parts of the human system, allowing us to function correctly.

The human form can interact with EMF/EMR because our own charged field acts as an antenna to this medium.

The World Health Organisation states:

"Electromagnetic fields affect us because our human bodies have their own electric and biochemical responses."

So we know that this technology influences us, but to what degree?

The WHO explains EMF as:

"Electric fields are created by differences in voltage: the higher the voltage, the stronger will be the resultant field. Magnetic fields are created when electric current flows: the greater the current, the stronger the magnetic field. An electric field will exist even when there is no current flowing. If current does flow, the strength of the magnetic field will vary with power consumption but the electric field strength will be constant". *[2]

Note how the electric field strength will be constant. This is important, as it means there is a continuation of pulsed energy communication, even when there is no current flowing. This tells us that an electromagnetic field is potentially affecting us if we are in the vicinity of the device's range, even when not in direct use.

There are many objects in the modern world that emit EMR such as: mobile phones, mobile phone masts, DECT cordless phones, baby monitors, computers, wireless console controllers, internet routers, Wi-Fi, microwave ovens, and fluorescent lighting.

---

2   * *(Extract from Electromagnetic fields published by the WHO Regional Office for Europe in 1999 (Local authorities, health and environment briefing pamphlet series; 32).*

All of these devices are considered to be breakthrough gadgets that most of us, I'm sure, would find it difficult to live without. It has become easier than ever to interact with each other via wireless technology almost anywhere on the planet.

Unfortunately, these devices emit radiation which can damage our DNA even from what is considered low exposure, in turn, creating a rise of new illnesses for a 21st century society. There have been many biased studies committed to the short-term adverse reactions of wireless technology but very few for possible long-term health effects. The telecommunications industry was allowed to market mobile phone usage to all ages without the need for an unbiased and independent scientific study on public health impacts before initiating widespread use. We were, and still are, the experiment.

The wireless network was released upon us and embraced by all without consumers knowing the full implications of radiation-emitting devices upon the body. The limited studies carried out were on short-term impacts and, ultimately, based on flawed data.

No sooner than funding for research on health impacts began, the bias toward industry favour was initiated. Following the money trail for funding of studies will often lead you to direct conflicts of interest.

Dr. Henry Lai, a University of Washington Scientist in Cellular and Molecular Engineering, carried out a review of 85 papers on the damaging effects of DNA from microwave radiation coming from mobile phones. 75% of the studies performed that showed no effects on human health were funded by the wireless industry or the military-industrial complex.

Our current mainstream scientific data about safety is over 17 years old and is largely based on studies that had been carried out regarding the thermal heating of tissue while using such devices, known as non-ionising radiation. Because such little heat is emitted when in use, it was widely accepted that wireless technology posed no danger to humans. What was either not taken into account or avoided in studies were the "non-thermal" effects, of which are being proved to cause damage to life. The industry, in its majority, still stands by the old data as it fits well with their profit margins, while more and more independent studies are claiming with growing evidence that *"non-thermal"* effects are significantly more dangerous than we were led to believe.

"There's enough science to suggest that cell phone radiation can cause cancer, but not enough political will to implement measures to reduce exposure. We're setting ourselves up for an epidemic of cancers in the future that should be preventable based on the knowledge we have now. If you use a cell phone and hold it to your head, the cancers you see elevated are brain cancer, tumours of the auditory nerve, tumours of the parotid gland, the salivary gland and the cheek right by the ear." -David Carpenter, MD Professor, Environmental Health Sciences, and Director, Institute for Health and the Environment, School of Public Health, University of Albany.

It is in my opinion that the mobile phone and wireless industry have been allowed to generate billions and manipulate the dangers facing society in favour of huge contracts that have made many corporate entities very wealthy, while ignoring the dangers that were discovered decades ago and keeping silent. Telecommunications is now one of the largest industries on the planet which has changed the face of Earth with a potential invisible death. It has such power amongst political ties now that its lobbying power is never denied, and far too much is at stake for it to admit to any inconsistencies in its laudable studies or any legitimate current findings regarding EMF/EMR safety issues. The growth within telecommunications has been enormous, a global swathe of mobile masts sprouting out of every corner of our landscape and Wi-Fi in nearly all public areas with 4 billion users connecting magically via a disrupted ether. Our airspace is forever changed and charged in a way that our bodies were never designed to cope with so rapidly although, from evolutionary changes in radiation protection from the sun, we have no natural defence against such a bombardment of unnatural digital frequencies, and children of the digital age may face far worse consequences in the years to come. Our cells react to this unseen attack, showing confusion under analysis and by slowing their processes, leading to a hindrance of our protective immune system. We expose ourselves to this technology 24/7, even at night when we need quality uninterrupted sleep to repair our daytime damage. Wireless connections are constantly pulsing digital frequencies when switched on and not even in use. Wi-Fi, and other wireless devices, can deplete melatonin and lead to poor sleep quality. A mobile phone can affect your cells at night if within 3 feet of your body, and so all devices should be switched off at night or at least moved to the other side of the room. It is ok to disconnect every night at least and give your body a break while it heals through rest and sleep.

"Science is one of the tools society uses to decide health policy. In the case of telecommunications equipment, such as cell phones, wireless networks, cell phone antennas, PDAs, and portable phones, the science is being ignored". -Professor Havas, Trent University

Mobile phone use is reportedly affecting sperm count within males; carrying a phone in your pocket for 4 hours a day can reduce sperm productivity. As male sperm is far more vulnerable than female eggs, men are experiencing more mutations as a result of radiating devices, so perhaps in the years to come all men may become completely infertile and reproduction will follow a course of clinical intervention for anyone wishing to have children? The public health issues associated with the use of wireless data transmission in the world today are being overlooked and, as yet, the safety parameters in place are simply inadequate. The indiscriminate nature of this technology is extremely worrying and should be of great concern, especially in public buildings and spaces. Our rapid adaption to such a way of living for so many is having consequences, not only for adverse health reactions but by quickly escalating into an image/status accessory to match. We are led to believe that we need these devices, that we cannot live without them, and that our street credibility is dearly affected for not having the latest smartphone. For a technology that is being used to increase communication links 24/7 wherever you may be, I feel we have lost the ability to deal with each other on a human level, learning expressions, tone, and how to build trust collectively as we have done for thousands of years. Nowhere is this more apparent than how the newest generation of children have become digital addicts, succumbing to a cognitive dissonance instead of a tangible engagement with the world and its people. There is an anxiety attachment to these digital devices that I see in adults and children alike, which is leading us to secondary health concerns that, over time, may transpire into an increasing epidemic.

Albert Einstein once said:

"I fear the day that technology will surpass our human interaction. The world will have a generation of idiots."

Perhaps many that read this can already see where this could take society and may have also witnessed this insistent technology take over the human race. We were sold this idea without ever being given full disclosure of safety; is it really necessary that we are connected to some digital force 24/7, 365 days of the year? I mean, who is really that important that you cannot switch off for at least a few hours a day?

There is little doubt we are being exposed to low levels of damaging radiation and harmful frequencies from telecommunications, and there is too much independent evidence to simply turn a blind eye.

There are many professional individuals that have the capacity to recognise a problem with wireless technology, and each has committed a great deal of time and experience in exposing this invisible threat using validated and well-researched data.

The current safety levels provided by ICNIRP (the International Commission on Non-Ionizing Radiation Protection) are far from adequate, or even accurate, considering the wealth of research available with very different conclusions to what we are all adhering to.

It is exceptionally difficult to understand, at first, the possibility that industry does not have our well-being as a primary and unbiased objective before mass production yet, even the organisations, institutes, and agencies that are in place apparently protecting society from danger of manufactured goods are really providing an incapable effort to do so with all the resources at our disposal on Earth.

Barrie Trower, an English gentleman and scholar, advises people all over the globe of microwave radiation dangers. He has extensive naval experience with this technology and in his own words:

"Unlike medication where there is a safe level for children, there is no safety level for microwave radiation for children, not one. I have never ever seen a single scientist brave enough to produce a safety level of microwave radiation for a child. There isn't one that exists. Children do not have our immune systems they are not developed. Their bones are soft, the microwaves penetrate very easily. Inside

their bones they are producing stem cells which make their immune systems and all other parts of their body. Their skulls are thin and children absorb more radiation because they are smaller and nearer the wavelength, so they act as aerials."

The long-term effects of low-level radiation for our children could have a huge impact on our future generation's health if no immediate changes occur, and could be similar to our society today, looking back regarding the dangers of smoking on a population. We know so much about the dangers of smoking now but didn't for so many years while we were sold the benefits of smoking by doctors of the early 20th century.

It is my opinion that in 20-30 years' time, microwave radiation will be far worse than smoking ever was, because of its indiscriminate and invisible touch upon all who are within its reach. Let's face it; it happens to be almost anywhere public, and even upon children and unborn foetuses within the comfort of your own home. I fear that, as this will be occurring collectively, we may not even recognise the far-reaching implications of our new digital prisons.

By far the most vulnerable sector of our wider society is that of children and pregnant women carrying life. Women are unaware of the imminent dangers posed to their developing foetuses while using smartphones; this action of free use by mothers and all humans has now become so ingrained within our daily activities that, by the time mass knowledge of these dangers emerges, it may be too late. A new generation of children is already being born into a digitally-bombarded atmosphere which is slowing the integral building blocks of their health and learning. The slowing and damaging production of mitochondrial DNA that happen to be the building blocks of a forming body is the unseen danger lurking within our devices, as there has already been links to autism, ADD, ADHD and higher incidences of leukaemia in families living close to mobile masts. Electromagnetic hypersensitivity is growing amongst people as another symptom associated to overexposure of harmful microwaves.

"To many EMR researchers, a pregnant woman chatting on her iPhone, or resting a Blackberry, or laptop, on her ample abdomen, appears as shocking as seeing her smoking or drinking alcohol. The new health warning during pregnancy: refrain from drugs, alcohol, tobacco, prolonged proximity to electric devices, and avoid mobile technology. As with tobacco, and other public health issues, there's usually a long time lag between people getting sick and governments taking action, as we mentioned. Not only are the agencies in charge not stepping in to fund needed research and provide necessary precautions, most are still defending the existing 'safe' levels which respected scientists warn are not protecting us. Meanwhile, reports from the European Union alert us that childhood brain cancers are on the rise." - An extract from Kerry Crofton's 'A Wellness Guide for the Digital Age'

The conclusions from current independent research are too slowly becoming a turning point for scientific and public awareness, as it is this awareness that will help implement the needed safety warnings in order to prevent an entire generation of new illnesses. We need to demand, from authorities, the right to challenge the existing safety guidelines. It is my hope that this happens as prevention rather than an unfolding future problem, where finding cures or offering treatment for neurologically-damaged people becomes yet another lucrative industry.

The greatest action we can take to empower ourselves is to limit the use of Wi-Fi in the home and get your internet hard-wired using Ethernet cables. Remove cordless phones. Cook proper dinners and recycle your microwave, as these devices destroy the nutrients in your food. Create an environment, especially for your young ones, where a night's rest is not interrupted by electromagnetic disturbance. Simple steps are effortless to make and yet will serve the health and well-being of all members of the family. As with all the information printed here, it is important to get over the initial shock and anger swiftly and easily take responsible action to change small things that can have big impacts on your family life. The reported damage caused by overexposure to wireless technology is a well-known phenomenon to those with skilled backgrounds who were ultimately willing to question accepted truths.

You can hire an Acoustimeter online to determine if you have elevated levels that could be affecting your family home. These are interesting devices which can show you what you cannot see with your eyes.

Within the next 2 years, the UK will see a nationwide roll-out of smart meters that have Wi-Fi capability, and leading the way is a gas giant who has installed 2 million already into homes and businesses. These devices monitor your electrical use and are being promoted as a money-saving, time-saving, fully-interactive gizmo that will bring ease and comfort to the streamlining of energy use within the home or business, and essentially save us all money off our bills.

The issues are the savings heralded by energy companies that will not readily be passed onto consumers, where we could save better by simply switching tariff and turning our heating down a degree or two. The estimated cost of £11billion is a whopping investment that is inevitably indirectly passed back to the consumer, with such tactics of selling to the public having been used again and again. Certainly, government-backed initiatives historically fall flat of their intended costs and benefits, yet we continue to fall for it because we are not exposing our perceptions to the potential hazards which are ignored and never disclosed. We also need to realise this is not our fault and that, for a very long time, society has been fed incorrect information.

So far, Generation 1 smart meters have had a lot of concerns, with reports of inferior machines and poor programming leading many customers' meters reverting back to analogue when switching suppliers. What is even more astonishing is the EU directive for energy supply compliance that can issue fines against energy companies that are not fulfilling quotas of installations. Penalties exist even though it is known that inadequate machines are being installed and that health concerns have been documented, with the industries promoting their safety also being misled by inaccurate science, but we are still the experiment. Having a smart meter in your home is the equivalent of bringing a mobile phone mast into your space; the adverse reactions reported on the prolonged exposure of smart meters is increasing and scandalous, especially for a high number of Americans who been affected by electromagnetic sensitivity and also those which have reported energy companies forcefully installing meters into people's homes without permission.

Dramatically, this has largely been ignored or not adequately investigated by all institutes and organisations set with the task of either concern or profit. A device like this is capable of producing a pulsed frequency throughout your home or business space 24 hours a day; we know not only from the information given here but by the plethora of evidence showing us that this technology is not anywhere near as safe as we are led to believe. The International BioInitiative report paints a very different picture in its findings and only further confirms that Wi-Fi is harmful, especially to children.

"What is clear is that the existing public safety standards limiting these radiation levels in nearly every country of the world look to be thousands of times too lenient". - 2007 BioInitiative Report

The only mechanism preventing the clarity of such information spreading into mainstream knowledge is the unpopular conclusions we can draw from them, but they are not an accepted truth so they are discarded from view and debate. The energy companies give us a poor deal considering the viable solutions that could be implemented which does not affect our privacy rights or health, and which could be far more in-keeping with 21st century engineering. Of course, everyone has the right to refuse the installation of a smart meter, yet it is important to understand why not to have one in your home in the first place, so educate yourself.

Technology has captured our imaginations for decades - as has the digital phenomenon that has either been an intruder or saviour to many in society - and we have learnt to accept, without question, the assimilation of mobile communication into our every living hour. It is time to dispute the claims of safety for the sake of our children so that they may experience an environment that is not as invisibly polluted as we are today.

Chapter 6

Vaccination: Fear, Myth and Belief

Vaccination is big business and big money for doctors, drug companies, and the government, but vaccines are by no means proven safe, as we are being led to believe.

The statement above is in direct conflict with what we continue to be told by GPs, the mainstream medical community, and the controlled media network supported by government. Nearly all parents I speak to have absolutely no idea what is actually in a vaccine, and nearly all of my living life neither did I. I didn't really care, I mean, why should I? For as long as I can remember, I have been told that I need a certain vaccine to prevent the body from succumbing to ill health or premature death, especially childhood diseases, and that I must be vaccinated so I can lead a healthy life. Repeatedly, I was told that I must let doctors stick this needle in me and subsequently my children too. Repetition is a key tactic in dissolving historical significances from view and enabling mainstream observers to follow the current trend in popular information. When global markets have such a deep interest in the health of a nation, a breeding platform can arise for fraudulent activity to occur that progressively breaks down the action of critical thinking.

I, like many others, started researching what was in the ingredients of a vaccine and whether they have any benefit toward the strengthening of our immune systems. What I found was shocking, and helped me to try and understand how such a fraud can be in existence for a 21st century society allegedly committing proper and correct science. Through fear, we are led to believe that our immune systems are not capable of tackling threats from outside the body, and we are also led to believe that vaccination is the only proven scientific way of protecting the body from certain diseases.

Our decisions regarding the allowance of injecting foreign materials into our body are mostly based on fear and not fact, and therefore the vaccine industry has become an increasingly lucrative lifetime procedure. What we believe to be facts are more often than not based on manipulated scientific data. Most of what we believe to be true is merely a fabrication of a repeater simply repeating what is dictated to them. Influenced and biased studies become accepted as truth and then lies become accepted mainstream procedure for all to follow.

Most doctors could not even tell you what is in a vaccine. Try it; obtain the ingredient information for a single vaccine from the internet (check its validity) and quiz your doc. We are being sold a great lie through our ignorance, which is being perpetrated by, yet again, the mega corporation which dictates its policies, recommendations, and strategic agenda for eradicating any opposition. The very organisations that are supposed to be protecting our human rights go along with the inaccuracies conjured up by these giants, and any questioning against the validity of such claims is always drowned in fake science and clever PR marketing.

One Canadian physician, Dr. Guylaine Lanctot, puts it this way:

"The medical authorities keep lying. Vaccination has been an assault on the immune system. It actually causes a lot of illnesses. We are actually changing our genetic code through vaccination. . .100 years from now we will know that the biggest crime against humanity was vaccines."

Australian researcher, Dr Viera Scheibner PhD, also explains that:

"It is a well-documented fact that the incidence and mortality from infectious diseases fell by 90% well before any vaccine was even introduced... So [the U.S.] mandated vaccination and it resulted in a three-fold increase in whooping cough..."

"After a careful consideration of the history of vaccination gleaned from an impartial and comprehensive study of vital statistics, and

pertinent data from every reliable source, and after an experience derived from having vaccinated 31,000 subjects, I am firmly convinced that vaccination cannot be shown to have any logical relation to the diminution of cases of smallpox. Vaccination does not protect, it actually renders its subjects more susceptible by depressing the vital power and diminishing the natural resistance, and millions of people have died of smallpox which they contracted after being vaccinated" -J.W. Hodge MD in his book "The Vaccination Superstition"

"My data proves that the studies used to support immunisation are so flawed that it is impossible to say if immunisation provides a net benefit to anyone or to society in general. This question can only be determined by proper studies which have never been performed. The flaw of previous studies is that there was no long term follow up and chronic toxicity was not looked at. The American Society of Microbiology has promoted my research...and thus acknowledges the need for proper studies." -John B.Classen, M.D., M.B.A.

Vaccines cause inflammation and can be immunosuppressive, meaning they can suppress an immune system which may not return to normal for days or weeks.

The components used in vaccines are neurotoxic and may cause brain and immune dysfunction. These components can include heavy metals, preservatives, and aluminium adjuvants. Vaccines introduce large foreign molecules into the body, which induces an inflammatory response to stimulate antibodies. However, if your body responds to these foreign molecules in a way that causes a type of inflammation that does not resolve itself, severe allergies can develop and pave the way for illness and autoimmune diseases.

The major ingredients vaccines are composed of which should be an immediate concern to any adult or parent are heavy metals. There is a huge social stigma associated with those parents wishing not to vaccinate their children and my heart goes out to those who have the courage to stand up to misguided perceptions which have fully erect egos, yet are not willing to commit time into research and almost always are so easily willing to condemn without investigation. Parents of vaccinated children are taught to be fearful of children that have not been vaccinated and are generally despondent at those parents choosing a different path to the rest of popular conformity, but we need to recognise the PR campaigns put forth by the media on behalf of corporations and their business interests. The supposed scientific facts are still being controlled using fraudulent activity and the reliance of a fear, myth, and belief-based society. That is what Big Pharma relies on; that we are too busy with our socially-engineered working lives to even contemplate those pressing matters we need to question. If my child has not been vaccinated, how on Earth can they pose any kind of risk toward a vaccinated child? They have been vaccinated, so then surely they are protected from this threat my child may pose? And if my child has a healthy diet with a strong immune system, why should they be categorised as an unprotected threat?

We should become aware that most diseases from the 19th and 20th centuries were already in massive decline prior to vaccines being introduced for specific illness. Vaccine companies have used edited snippets of data from a much shorter chronological timeline to create the appearance that injecting humans drastically reduced childhood diseases. This is simply not true when you understand the forgotten history of Westernised illness in the last 150 years.

It is difficult to contemplate such a barbaric idea for combating disease and how it has become normal practice when we familiarise ourselves with Vaccine history. There are very revealing books and documentaries on this subject and, in order to gain a grounded opinion, many should be read and watched to understand the subject completely and we should not simply rely on what the media feeds us now.

Flu shots are a winter drug bonanza for flu vaccine companies. GBI Research notes there's a $2.9 billion market riding on seasonal flu vaccines. The importance for these companies to introduce further recommendations and greater power to vaccinate those who are willing and ready to believe in the fear is crucial to escalating profit margins. Their easiest option is to vaccinate all, like mass herd immunity. This is nothing short of medical fraud, as there are no proven facts to confirm efficacy and acceptance is entirely based on misinformation. Look at how blackmail is being used today to make employees succumb to a flu vaccine in hospitals; to use the threat of losing your job is insane and a clear and concise attack against both your human rights and civil liberties for the right to reject mass immunisation. If we continue to sit on the fence and turn the other cheek while many suffer, then this tyranny will be mandated again in all industry within the UK, along with already being introduced in the US and Australia by force. The lies about vaccines have become an embarrassment to doctors and are deceiving new students into believing vaccines immunise. Synthetic introduction of toxic chemicals has never, can never, and will never give lifelong immunity even with boosters, because you can still contract whatever it is the schedule is trying to vaccinate you against. So, if vaccines do not offer full prevention and protection of your immune system, then why do we become pin cushions so readily? The lifetime return for booster vaccines is down to the fact that all vaccines have a very short effective time span, which is contrary to the original projections for many inoculations, which was discovered very early on in vaccine history. So, instead of creating new energy to increase life and prevent illness efficiently, we are made to return, like an addict to a dealer. This is diabolical economics for us and the dealers are always rubbing their hands together. Researching for yourself can be empowering, as so much of our reality is based on manipulated data to benefit only one winner and I can assure you, it's not us. Big Pharma have fallen far short of their predicted claims. The forgotten history of how vaccines came into existence is a stern reality check of indisputable data that will lead anyone to question all current vaccine mainstream myth. Corporations cannot patent a carrot or a Brazil nut or any food to make us well from illness. Only synthesised matter can be issued a patent for profit protection, enabling market domination for drug producers. So, here we are, having tea with the Mad Hatter mega corporations, but are we being denied a simple resolution? Their tea has become an elixir of untruths and is proving very costly to the lives of those that have proven vaccine damage as a result of recommended, or forced, injections. There are many cases in which people have been paid to go away quietly and sign gagging orders. The National Vaccine Injury Compensation Program (VICP) has paid out over $1 billion in court case settlements; many cases go unreported by mainstream media and, all too often, access to medical records is limited or information blocked from investigation.

Avoiding a serious case of the flu is not an arduous task; by following simple guidelines, you can keep your immune system operating at an optimum for any age.

Optimise your vitamin D levels. In the winter, we receive less sunlight and even less motivation to go outside to get the sunlight we need when it is shining. Vitamin D is crucial in protecting our bodies, and it is only produced by our skin when it is exposed to sunlight. It is thought that this deficiency throughout winter is making us ill. Think about it; we are all less ill in the summer. Vitamin D is found in very few foods and in very low concentrations, which proves how important healthy exposure to the sun's rays is for humans. Failing to gain sun exposure, it is important to take a vitamin D3 supplement. Vitamin D is responsible for regulating calcium metabolism, bone health, cell growth, and the protection of the immune system. Avoid sugar and processed foods, get enough rest, commit to regular exercise, and take a good source of omega-3 and 6 fats (hempseed oil is the best suited to humans). Washing your hands prevents the spread of a virus to your nose, mouth, or other people, and using natural antibiotics - such as colloidal silver, oil of oregano, garlic, and olive leaf extract - are far more effective than any flu jab.

"Historical data shines a great light upon the darkness of men who in their ignorance led us all to believe it was safe to become injected with a poison."

In 1940, there were 857 deaths in the UK from measles [3]. By 1967, the year before the measles vaccine was introduced, the figure had dropped to 99 deaths in 27 years of no vaccine. 11 years prior to this, in 1956, it was as low as 28. The UK in 1967 saw a progressive reduction of measles-related deaths to less than one eighth of the total figure back in 1940; this occurred due to better living environments, sanitation, and with no vaccine. Back in 1968, when a measles vaccine was introduced through careful timing, it appeared that this vaccine over the course of the next 20 years was the main factor in the reduction of measles deaths and notifications. The vaccine companies and governments insisted it was their chemical product that lead to its rapid decline amongst the population, but the decline was already in massive free-fall before 1968 and we can only speculate where such figures would be, had no corporate entity appear to come to our rescue and obscure an existing decline for decades. An interesting study was carried out in 2002; a randomised controlled trial (a gold standard of scientific research) was performed by Dr. Stephen P. Luby in Karachi, Pakistan. The goal of the study was to assess the impact of hand washing and bathing with soap in settings where infectious diseases are leading causes of childhood disease and death. The study became known as the Karachi Health Soap Study. Just by simply introducing anti-bacterial and plain soap into 25 neighbourhoods where disease was rife, dramatic results followed. After a 51 week period, there was 52% less diarrhoea and 50% less pneumonia. [4] Hygiene can play an important role in combatting illness by keeping the first level of defence operating at its optimum using self-awareness, education, and common sense. Our sanitation infrastructure has been the primary force by which disease has dissipated, but the large scale installation of sanitary means into cities in the Western world is never credited or associated to the rapid decline of deaths and illness prior to vaccines being introduced. We should be thanking the intuitive brilliance of Victorian engineering and the plumbers who changed the face of daily living from putrid walkways into clean streets.

A study, published in Human and Experimental Toxicology - a peer-reviewed journal indexed by the National Library of Medicine - studied over 38,000 reports of infant hospitalisations and deaths following vaccinations. They reported statistically significant relationships between the number of vaccine doses administered to infants and infant hospitalisation and mortality rates.

Infants who received 2 vaccines simultaneously were significantly less likely to be hospitalised than infants who received 3 or more vaccines at the same time. Infants who received 3 vaccines simultaneously were significantly less likely to be hospitalised than infants who received 4 or more vaccines at the same time. Babies who received 6, 7, or 8 vaccines during a single paediatric well-baby visit were the most likely to be hospitalised following their injections. This concluded that the hospitalisation rate increased linearly from 11.0% for infants receiving 2 vaccine doses to 23.5% for infants receiving 8 vaccine doses.

Dr. Gary Goldman and Neil Z. Miller, authors of the study, also discovered that younger infants were significantly more likely to be hospitalised after receiving vaccinations than older infants. In addition, infants who received 5-8 vaccines simultaneously were significantly more likely to die following their shots than infants who received 1-4 vaccines simultaneously. [5]

Vaccine companies individually test their drugs but, to date, there have been no studies carried out on the safety of combining many vaccines administered in one go. 2, 4, and 6 month old babies are expected to receive vaccines for polio, hepatitis B, diphtheria, tetanus, pertussis, rotavirus, Haemophilus influenzae type B, and pneumococcal, all during a single well-baby visit even though this combination of 8 vaccines was never tested in clinical trials. The toxicity of these drugs increase 10 fold and in some cases many times more when given together instead of a single vaccination.

Dr. Harold Buttram also stated:

"It is universally recognized among toxicologists that combinations of toxic chemicals may bring exponential increases in toxicity; that is, two toxic chemicals in combination will bring a ten-fold or even a hundred-fold increase in toxicity. A classical example of this principle was the Schubert study in which it was found that the amount of lead and the amount of mercury, when each was given separately, would be lethal for one percent of rats tested, would become lethal for one hundred percent of rats tested when combined. In vaccines this principle would apply at least to mercury and aluminium, both

of which are potent neurotoxins."

Although we are encouraged to have vaccines by health authorities that protest about potential and existing outbreaks of virus and disease, we are still not informed about the potential side-effects that such vaccines have on a human body and, when you consider that in the UK in 2010 there were 374 reported cases of measles in a population of over 60 million people, we are talking about a risk factor of less than 0.001%! Mumps, measles, and rubella can leave victims paralysed and can be fatal, but the overwhelming majority of us are capable of fighting off disease with the healthy support of a strong immune system. For a less than 0.1% chance of even contracting such illnesses, it seems highly out of place to use synthetic vaccines, knowing there are so many associated side-effects being reported globally. Large drug companies have made, and continue to make, secret compensation pay-outs to damaged victims and yet none of this is brought to the table when parents and individuals make their choices. Informed decisions are our inalienable rights to a healthy life and, while some of us may need protection from higher selected governance, there are still so many others who do not. It is this simple indifference that continues to divide opinion and sees it becoming more like a single science religion with a medical community believing that their way is the only way and that those who stand up and ask questions are wrong, even despicably so. In my opinion, there is always more than one way to achieve an end goal and, while targets on scales such as population disease control are no easy feat, we should embrace diet sustained ways at reducing health problems and allow an easier, less prejudice platform for those to speak about their findings, even if they do affect the status quo of drug companies. Vaccines combined create toxic overload inside the body and it is the way our bodies react to these foreign toxins that dictate whether we reject them or live with them building up in our form. Where are the long-term studies proving vaccine safety? Most healthy bodies have the ability to ward off most incoming attacks, and even when the body does succumb it reprograms itself, learning to heal at a natural and acutely responsive pace. We can help this process by following simple guidelines incorporated into our daily lives. We, as a species, need to defend our rights to humanity and be rightfully free to question single science policies from corporations, who came like a thief in the night and stripped us of our knowledge.

The reason I feel it's important to mention vaccines is that the CDC (Center for Disease Control) admitted, on its own website, that between 10 and 30 million Americans were infected with the SV-40 Virus in polio vaccines, which has been found in certain types of Cancer. Although it has not been determined that SV-40 had caused the Cancers, I believe this issue is more about accountability and the avoidance of responsibility when things go wrong in the name of modern science. I firmly believe that we are polluting the bodies of babies with foreign materials and heavy metals that are not biologically compatible with us. Overloading under developed human life with toxins could be the first steps at creating the environment within for Cancer to multiply. We should question why so many young children have cancers and auto-immune diseases. Are we falling before we have even learnt to walk?

Chapter 7
Herbs, the Lost Knowledge

Herbs have played an intrinsic part in history toward the treatment of many conditions the world over. Human beings, for centuries, used what grew from the Earth to help heal and ward off infection. How else do you think we came this far before the advent of pharmaceuticals?

Records indicate that humans have been studying herbal remedies for over 5000 years. It was the Sumerians who were perhaps among the first at recording various medical uses, and some of the plants which they described were thyme, caraway, and laurel. Every known civilisation since Ancient Sumer has provided evidence for the use of herbs, but most notably, India and China. When the Celts were prevalent in Great Britain, herbal medicine was provided by their intellectual leaders, Druids.

Druids had immense knowledge of the land that was passed down through generations of study on a verbal memory basis as they allowed nothing to be written; this, I suspect, protected the preservation of such knowledge. Invading Romans, at the same time, brought with them further knowledge from the Egyptians and Greeks. Even before their invasion of Britain, they had sent green-fingered parties over the Channel to sow many varieties of herbs and seeds in preparation of their future life here in Britain. It is only in very recent times chronologically that mainstream consensus has frowned upon the evidence of herbs curing common ailments and disease. Thankfully, there are many studies emerging that are backing the validity of what many already know to be true. Tinctures, teas, infusions, and decoctions can all be made safely at home with minimum cost. There are hundreds of books on how to use herbs safely, how to grow them yourself, when to harvest them, what to look for, and what to avoid. The list is really endless considering the amount of herbs with different properties in our world, and it doesn't take long to understand how to use them. Most common herbs are very easy to grow in your garden, especially lavender, rosemary, thyme, sage, mint, camomile, feverfew, peppermint, oregano, bay, and basil. All of the herbs mentioned are not only great for culinary use, but have particular properties that help the body.

Below is a short list of known uses and benefits from herbs:

Thyme: Antibacterial, antifungal, antiseptic.
Sage: Antiseptic, blood sugar normaliser, improves memory, uplifting.

Lavender: Helps balance emotions, induces peaceful sleep, increases cell renewal.
Rosemary: Antioxidant, boosts blood circulation, enhances memory, eases muscles.
Oregano: Excellent immune booster, antioxidant, antibacterial.
Camomile: Restful sleep, menstrual cramps, IBS, wound healing.
Basil: Antibacterial, treat constipation, stomach cramps and indigestion as well as cold, flu, asthma, whooping cough, bronchitis and sinus infections.

There is an abundance of wild grown herbs that, with a little study, can be utilised and harvested for nothing. Studies performed recently on rosemary for improving memory are another step closer toward proving what many folk have understood to work without the need for science to tell us so. Whilst adding weight to the benefits of the humble rosemary and its uses as a possible dementia aid, we should be, at the very least, demanding these simple remedies to be readily available to us.

Even though herbs have superior properties for human well-being in nourishment and healing, mainstream medical views look at them with a lack of understanding and see them as inferior toward our fight against health problems with a 20th century mind-set. Again, profitability is the cause of these herbs never really showing their true colours in the greater society; they elude the minds of pro-Pharma drug enthusiasts, and it is their simple effectiveness that has been kept from mainstream treatment. Offering humanity natural but potent remedies enables us, as a whole, to become more aware of how important this world is and what it has to offer us in healing and restorative value.

One great example of herbs curing disease is that of Rene Caisse, a Canadian Nurse, who was well-documented for providing herbal cures against cancer. In 1922, Rene Caisse happened to notice some scar tissue on the breast of an elderly English woman. The woman said that doctors had diagnosed her with breast cancer years before. However, the woman didn't want to risk surgery nor did she have the money for it. The English woman had met an old Indian medicine man in the 1890s who told her that he could cure her cancer with herbal tea. The woman took the medicine man's advice, and consequently was still alive nearly thirty years later to pass on this herbal remedy to Nurse Caisse. In 1924, she decided to test the tea on her aunt who had cancer of the stomach and was given about six months to live. Her aunt lived for another 21 years, cancer-free. Rene Caisse (pronounced "Reen Case") later gave the tea to her 72-year old mother who was diagnosed with inoperable cancer of the liver, with only days to live. Her mother recovered and lived without cancer for another 18 years.

In the coming years, Caisse perfected the original medicine man's formula, testing various herbs on laboratory mice and human cancer patients.

She eventually reduced the tea to four herbs: burdock root, sheep sorrel, slippery elm, and turkey rhubarb. She named the formula Essiac, which is her surname spelled backwards. Rene Caisse devoted over fifty years of her life to treating hundreds of cancer patients with Essiac. So effective were her treatments that, in 1938, her supporters gathered 55,000 signatures for a petition, amongst other petitions, to allow Rene Caisse to continue treating cancer patients. A bill was introduced in the Ontario legislature to (allegedly) "authorise Rene Caisse to practice medicine in the Province of Ontario in the treatment of cancer and conditions therein". Due to the machinations of the medical establishment, the bill failed to pass by just three votes. Rene Caisse operated her cancer clinic under the supervision and observation of a number of doctors. Based on what those doctors saw with their own eyes, eight of them signed a petition to the Department of National Health and Welfare at Ottawa, asking that Nurse Caisse be given facilities to do independent research on her discovery. Their petition, dated at Toronto on October 27, 1926, read as follows:

To Whom It May Concern:

"We the undersigned believe that the 'Treatment for Cancer' given by Nurse R.M. Caisse can do no harm and that it relieves pain, will reduce the enlargement and will prolong life in hopeless cases. To the best of our knowledge, she has not been given a case to treat until everything in medical and surgical science has been tried without effect and even then she was able to show remarkable beneficial results on those cases at that late stage." We would be interested to see her given an opportunity to prove her work in a large way. To the best of our knowledge she has treated all cases free of any charge and has been carrying on this work over the period of the past two years."

Initially, Rene was not aware of the control that the medical/pharmaceutical establishment had over governments. After the petition was delivered to the National Health and Welfare Department, she was continually threatened with arrest until she finally withdrew from public view. Unlike Nurse Caisse, the medical establishment was more interested in making money than in helping people. Essiac was cheap. It could cut into the lucrative profits from radiation, chemotherapy, and surgery treatments that often do more harm than good. Essiac is non-toxic. Rene said, "Chemotherapy should be a criminal offence." Dr. Ralph Moss was appointed to the Cancer Advisory Panel that evaluates alternative cancer therapies for the government. On his website and in his book entitled 'Cancer Therapy', Dr. Moss points out that each of the herbs in Essiac has been scientifically shown to contain anti-cancer substances. The scepticism surrounding herbal treatments are related to the limited and relative blackout of information for the beneficial uses of plant life. Since humans first walked the Earth, a symbiotic relationship existed between nature, us, and her gifts, and she has always provided the answers to our ailments. As herbs and natural remedies are no monetary equal to synthesised drugs, there simply is no reason for big corporations who own the media to report on them. Simple business prevents that which threatens to compete against a highly lucrative market. So successful the current medical doctrine has become that we have become willing to accept mainstream patter as the indisputable truth with no other formidable unpopular evidence allowed to present its findings.

Chapter 8
Dis-ease

"Disease" - Oxford dictionary states:

"disorder of structure or function in a human, animal, or plant, especially one that produces specific symptoms or that affects a specific location and is not simply a direct result of physical injury."

The word 'disease' and its origins are stated as *"being Middle English in the sense 'lack of ease; inconvenience."* Diseases are certainly an inconvenience; if it is allowed to evolve, it fundamentally puts the body at a dis-ease.

This dis-ease in life is a stern warning to correct, remove toxins, and cleanse the form from which a disease can grow and dominate the individual. So, if a disease is a "dis-order of structure", is it possible to bring about order of structure by boosting the immune system so it may target mutated cells and dispel them? Although disease may affect a specific location, it is the whole body that needs to be treated; neglecting the rest of the body from any treatment as a point of view is a terrible lack of understanding that will never produce long-term sufficient results. Cancer has become one of the most feared manmade medical conditions in the modern world today. When you consider that 1 in 4 of us are statistically likely to create this disease ourselves, it becomes a real threat posing serious questions that need answering in a profit-free environment. Current trends in consuming nutrient-deficient foods and an excess of unhealthy products is certainly a major contributor to the chronic conditions we face today. We are now living in an oxygen-deprived world where environmental pollution is increasing and the limitations of hospital treatment today still seems to produce very unsuccessful long-term results. Cytotoxic Chemotherapy drugs reportedly help less than 10% of patients. In a 14 year study called "The Contribution of Cytotoxic Chemotherapy to 5-year Survival in Adult Malignancies". by Graeme Morgan, Robyn Ward and Michael Barton. Concluded that "Cytotoxic Chemotherapy only makes a minor contribution to cancer survival". Of the 22 malignancies researched in the study only a 2.3% average mean was attributable to the effectiveness of Chemotherapy. It must be pointed out that in the study testicular Cancer was as high as 41.8% and Hodgkin's disease at 35.8%.

Although, would you pay for a service that was only successful 41% of the time at best? There needs to be an urgent evaluation on the effectiveness of modern Cancer treatments, to include surgery and radiation.

I understand that radiation is known to cause cells to turn cancerous, so why are we offered treatments that are essentially poison for the body? And do we really need to resort to surgery? There is evidence stating that cancerous cells can further spread after a biopsy and surgery. A biopsy is normally undertaken to determine a diagnosis of condition, which includes part or whole removal of a tumour, and can also be done with needles; either a core needle biopsy or a fine needle aspiration. Tumours, by their very nature, are produced by your immune system to prevent the spreading of cancerous cells. When needles and surgical instruments remove samples, the rate of possible spread is increased so greatly that, in some cases, they can dislodge some cancer cells, either into the interstitial fluid where they are carried away to lymph nodes, or possibly into the veins draining the tissue where they enter the vascular tree and travel to the lungs. It is also possible to drag some cells along the needle track or along the surgical incision. Doctors are not using adequate enough technology to guarantee a 0% chance of spreading cells to other parts of the body. They cannot witness and follow the small cells in real time and accurately comment on whether a quarantine zone for psychopathic cancer cells has been fully contained, or maybe the porter left the kitchen door ajar for some to escape? We, as a population, are in awe of what surgeons can perform with their tools on us humans; the strain a body is under when facing disease is only accentuated by the additional energy needed to repair invasive treatment. Perhaps the use of supporting the existing immune system and strengthening it from within would be better suited for many facing disease. The use of only a full nutrient, vitamin rich diet and to include beneficial supplements is all that may be needed to help cure more effectively with minimal side effects compared to current primitive methods. How simple does this solution sound in a perpetually complex and scientifically confusing world that we live in?

This view of nil surgery is working, has worked, and will be the true future of treating disease and, more importantly, preventing it too. This method can also work alongside pharmaceutical treatment if need be and will only add benefit to the strength of the immune system as it undergoes a toxic attack from chemotherapy or radiation.

The full onslaught of current cancer and disease-related drugs that we are recommended and, in some cases, forcefully so by unethical court systems, opens a door to unnecessary suffering that does kill millions of sufferers annually due to the continuation of popular accepted truths - that there are no cures for cancer, period. The existing criteria for the term 'cure' used within mainstream medicine is a five year goal post; if you reach this and you're still alive, then you're deemed cured, so what happens from six years onwards? This figure seems to contradict the present and historical testimonies from our fellow humans that chose to take responsibility for their own actions. Many sufferers globally are witnessing exceedingly better results outside or alongside mainstream treatment in terms of longevity and quality of life, which is significantly important with healing of any description and certainly raises doubts with our health services, its policy makers, and influencers, of which there are far too many.

Our diagnostic capabilities have increased tenfold after billions of pounds have been spent in an attempt to alleviate health issues we witness daily. Yet we still have no conclusive answers for true cures in the mainstream or, better yet, the correct information about how to prevent cancer occurring in the first place. Since the early part of the last century, we have been fed the lie that an apparent cure is just around the corner. These tactically fraudulent lies have kept a dominating industry floating along rather comfortably in an unaccountable protection racket for the Pharma mega corps.

Doctors are forced to keep using toxic legal drugs in a blinded attempt to combat disease. It really is the doctors hope that their drugs will kill the disease before they kill you...

We must learn to understand for ourselves the importance of knowing! We should make it our business to educate the mind in every area of our lives, rather than leaving the responsibility of the unknown in someone else's hands just because a white coat is facing us. We have the capacity to take action ourselves and for ourselves; this is empowering and can assist in the healing process. I have heard many times about the description of cancer sufferers and how they are "cancer victims", as if there is an external force set upon them for which they have no identifiable control over. Cancer is a manmade result of what you yourself inhale, ingest, or as a direct result of your surrounding environment. There are obviously many forms but, essentially, cancer occurs when the correct environment for it to thrive is created within the body. Right now, your immune system is destroying potentially cancerous cells from mutating out of control. Cancerous cells can only gain a foothold if your immune system is not functioning properly, which is why the nurture of the body's defence mechanism is paramount in alleviating a dis-ease. This attitude is overlooked in conventional wisdom and the best we are offered are mediums that systematically destroy the only thing trying to save us. All cancers need the same environment to grow, which seems to be a common weakness that is continuously unnoticed or never mentioned. When a healthy cell has its oxygen levels reduced, it can turn cancerous as cancer cells only live in an environment that is low in oxygen.

Our diet is one of the main contributors that lead to disease and illness today and, by accepting this as our responsibility, it is possible to have greater clarity in the steps we can take to heal ourselves. Psychologically, the moment you hand over your power and responsibility to a doctor and allow yourself to become a patient under a third party, you immediately lose your inert healing powers that we all have, and I mean all. To remain positively in control of your own well-being has a hugely beneficial effect on your body. It is wasting time just being positive whilst not in control; we have only one true object in our possession and that is our own body. You are its master, so you must retain at the very least some of your power to commit an educated action that can help you directly whilst you spend weeks waiting for answers in hospital waiting rooms. There is current research being carried out regarding the use of the mind in a positive motive to help stimulate our natural response to threats.

The highest level of control for your health is your own body's management system; keep a car topped up with the correct oil and fuel, and fewer problems will arise. The same applies to the machine that is our body. An ingenious propaganda program against those professionals who speak out and the manipulation by pharmaceutical companies has landed us in this situation with no apparent answers. Doctors have to follow what is only available to them through pharmaceuticals, to deviate into unconventional methods other than outlined in textbooks. They themselves become a victim, face ridicule and loss of license, which has happened to many around the globe who uncover - or get to close to - a solution or produce one for replication. Fear controls not only a sufferer of cancer but also the well-intentioned human and yet misinformed professional who is legally allowed to treat you.

Do most doctors believe they are really doing all they can with the correct resources currently available to us? Or do they keep quiet for the sake of the rat race that drives and distracts us all? To put it simply, our doctors are being lied to by Big Pharma whose sole interest is to keep shareholders happy and prevent well-documented known cures from reaching public view.

A recent study in August 2012, reported in the journal Nature Medicine, discovered that chemotherapy inflicts more damage than good. The damage toward healthy cells triggers them to release a protein that prolongs and stimulates tumour growth, leading to an eventual resilience to future treatment. Known as WNT16B, scientists who performed the research say that this protein created from chemo treatment boosts cancer cell survival and is the reason that chemotherapy actually ends lives more quickly.

Co-author Peter Nelson of the Fred Hutchinson Cancer Research Center in Seattle explains:

"WNT16B, when secreted, would interact with nearby tumour cells and cause them to grow, invade, and importantly, resist subsequent therapy." [6]

"There is not one, but many cures for cancer available. But they are all being systematically suppressed by the ACS, the NCI and the major oncology centres. They have too much of an interest in the status quo." -Dr Robert Atkins, M.D.

"No medical man during his student days is taught to think. He is expected to assimilate the thoughts of others and to bow to authority. Throughout the whole of his medical career he must accept the current medical fashions of the day or suffer the loss of prestige and place. No public appointments, no coveted preferments are open to the medical man who declines to parrot the popular shibboleths of his profession."

Dr. Hadwen in his book 'The Difficulties of Dr. Deguerre' on why most doctors will accept and perpetuate the status quo in medical treatment, no matter how unsatisfying or unsuccessful.

There is a silence that seldom stirs into action. Doctors do not protest for fear of losing their income, and patients do not protest because belief and false trust in what doctors are doing is everything within their power to heal us. We all believe, with good faith and intentions, that the current treatment from mainstream allopathic doctors is the only viable choice, but are we not living in a world full of choices? Nothing should be excluded from correct scrutiny where a possibility could be a viable solution. Future cures for all illness will not lie in the hands of pharmaceutical companies, but in our decisions that we make today, along with the better understanding of how the system of artificial drug markets work and the affects their usage on humans has. The Earth can provide a vast number of useful resources that can cleanse the body from toxic overload without the need to absorb synthesised products created by folk in laboratories.

Annual UK costs for cancer treatment range from £5000-£35,000 respectively, depending on which drug is administered, the disease type, and other variables including availability and age-related life expectancy post-treatment. American medical figures can be larger due to the privatisation of health management. As an example of increased over-pricing of synthetic drugs, Substratum instantness - which is a chemotherapy drug manufactured by Roche for the treatment of HER2-positive breast cancer that has spread to other parts of the body - has a course of treatment which is a prohibitive £90,831. Needless to say, the NHS will not fund the use of this option. There would be no need to consider these explicit charges if health services were not dominated by industry. The cost of such medication is often prohibitive for nationalised health services to purchase, leaving many drugs unavailable to sufferers, which creates further frustration for an individual who is as much in the dark about disease solutions as their doctors.

2008 research puts the global economic impact of premature death and disability from cancer at $895billion worldwide. These staggering costs reflect the ineffectiveness of existing treatment programs. Much of this could be avoided if our scope to treat was broadened beyond synthetics and it is high time we collectively demanded the availability of other viable answers outside the box of limitations we are so trusting of.

If we continue to approach answers in a complex manner that never seem to address the root source of illnesses, we will simply add to the toll and business will carry on as usual.

What your doctor won't tell you:

Outlined below are several examples of how people and professionals have treated cancer, other than the methods that are currently available on the NHS. All the information below is considered controversial by the mainstream attitude, even though there is factual evidence to back up these procedures that still won't be acknowledged by a closed system.

To take part in any of these methods, I strongly suggest you do lots of reading to obtain as much information as possible before you think of trying these, consult your oncologist and GP, be open and honest, and simply ensure that what you are about to embark on causes you no harm. None of these methods require a degree to follow, and neither should they be reserved for only doctors to divulge. All medicine requires patience, respect, and time. Doctors are by their very oath supposed to teach us, and cause no harm to their patients, but this simple protocol is not adhered to. We speak of human rights relentlessly when war is waged upon poorer countries or upon animal welfare, so why not the conflict against human health success by the pharmaceutical network that is slowly strangling us from the inside out with their, what is essentially, poison for the body?

Cancer and other diseases are **anaerobic**, meaning they can only survive and thrive in areas that are low in oxygen. Viruses, bacteria, and pathogens are Anaerobic too.

All good bacteria inside of us are **aerobic**, meaning they flourish in areas of high oxygen.

Refined sugar will feed and increase mutated cell numbers.

High **acidic** environments caused by eating various types of foods enable disease to thrive.

Increasing the **alkalinity** of the body will aid greatly in eradicating illness.

Knowing this information about common weakness trends in disease would allow you to have a greater understanding about how you can also help yourself to combat illness. A first for chronic sufferers would be to change your diet and, if you can afford it, eat organic. Juice your vegetables and drink in the goodness of all the micronutrients your body is so desperately screaming out for. By juicing, you are basically doing all the hard work your body normally does to extract the vitamins that can help your immune system whilst fighting illness. Buy a good quality juicing machine, and then read and learn about vegetables and fruit and how amazing they can be for healing the body.

"When you cook the food, you lose 50% of the protein, 70-80% of the vitamins and minerals and close to 100% of the micronutrients." - Dr. Gabriel Cousins, M.D

It is known that by heating food to over 118 degrees you destroy much of the life-giving energy that your body requires. Even when we think we are eating healthily, I wonder how much true energy is left and makes it back out of the pan? Think about it. There are very low cases of disease in wild animals, why? Have you ever seen a lion whip out a grill and cook its kill? Every animal eats raw. I'm not suggesting we all commit to eating raw meat, yet it deserves thought as to how and why we heat our foods before consumption.

Look into raw vegetable diets, as they are proving to be exceptionally effective. Removing sugar from your diet slows the fermentation process your body performs as sugar is broken down where it helps feed disease. Caffeine and tea are best to avoid while healing.

Consulting your doctor whilst carrying out a juice fast will give you a clear idea of how your body is responding to such a change in diet, as your doctor can monitor your healing process. This can lead to a radical change in how you support your body through ill health; by taking responsibility for what you eat using knowledge of what foods heal. Who knows, you may teach your GP about the benefits of nutrition. Highly acidic food needs to be avoided, such as coffee (mentioned above also), alcohol, white or brown sugar, processed sea salt, cow's milk, artificial spreads, commercial cooking oil, refined bread and pasta containing gluten and, of course, dreaded processed foods. Eating lots of fresh vegetables and abstaining from red meat will help reduce an acidic environment to an alkaline one. Surprisingly, beans, lentils, peas, and pulses are higher in protein than most meats! Fresh fruit, seeds, unprocessed sea salt, herbal teas, cold pressed oils, natural butter, water, and exercise will help whilst combatting any illness and greatly reduce the time it takes you to heal.

Turmeric has been gaining immense scientific weight in recent years as being a superior natural anti-cancer spice. It is specifically the root of the turmeric plant which contains curcumin that scientists believe to be halting cancer. The best effects are against breast cancer, bowel cancer, stomach cancer, and skin cancer cells. A 2007 American study that combined curcumin with chemotherapy to treat bowel cancer cells in a laboratory showed that the combined treatment killed more cancer cells than the chemotherapy alone.

In another study regarding colon cancer by The Department of Surgery, Coalhouse University, Halifax, Nova Scotia, Canada, it was discovered that:

"Self-induced apoptosis" and *"Curcumin may therefore have*

therapeutic potential in the management of colon cancer, especially in tumours that are resistant to conventional chemotherapy."
Turmeric is cheap, effective, natural, and easily assimilated by the body.

Potentially, millions of pounds could be saved if this was given to patients instead of immune destroying chemo, or even as well as.

Barley grass and wheatgrass are also two things to look into, as many benefits are arising from taking these naturally alkaline supplements.

Vitamin B17 should be included if battling with disease, as this vitamin has been incredibly useful on every continent for centuries.

Dr. Ernst T. Krebs Jnr., a San Francisco biochemist, discovered in the 50s that cancers were a result of deficiencies in modern diets. He identified compounds originating from the nitride family, which are present in many forms of edible plant life.

For a far greater insight into this valuable vitamin, you should watch *"World without Cancer"* by G. Ed. Griffin.

Another interesting plant is the Graviola (Cannon suricate), or soursop. It is native to the Amazonian rainforest with its large and heart-shaped fruit; the leaf is packed with anti-cancer ingredients and has had a great deal of funding to synthesise its constituents. Millions were spent to try to replicate and then patent their efforts which ended all in vain, as the original could not be cloned. Several studies have been performed on the effectiveness of using Graviola to combat cancer cells. The National Cancer Institute performed the first scientific research in 1976. The results showed that the leaves and stems were found effective in attacking and destroying malignant cells. The results were published in an internal report and never released to the public.

A study published in the Journal of Natural Products conducted at the Catholic University of South Korea stated that one chemical was found to selectively kill colon cancer cells at *"10,000 times the potency of (the commonly used chemotherapy drug) Aureomycin..."*

The additional benefit of this plant is its ability to ONLY attack cancerous cells, leaving the rest of the body to cope as it should, resulting in no hair loss and a lack of the other devastating effects chemotherapy cause. It is known to effectively target and kill malignant cells in 12 types of cancer, including colon, breast, prostate, lung, and pancreatic. The leaf is rich in antioxidants called solanaceous acetogenic.

Ask yourself, why is it that we do not know about this fruit? Where are all the further studies on this plant, confirming its relevance to combat disease in the mainstream? Why is its use almost unheard of?

The most important thing to achieve with disease and its treatment is to bring the body into a natural oxygenated alkaline state and reduce toxicity, as disease finds it impossible to grow in these conditions. You must feed the body essential micronutrients that are found in fruit and vegetables and limit red meat. This can be a very hard change to implement, but what is harder; a change in diet, or letting family watch a loved one waste away on primitive treatment?

"Breathe, breathe in the air."

Remember to exercise; 15 minutes a day is all that may be needed. Meditation and yoga are not just for hippies and long bearded Indian swamis. Understand that your breath has a calming effect. Chaos in your environment while healing is of no benefit and can worsen the impact of illness. A slower pace of life and learning to breathe correctly will help with both mental and physical aspects of any human beings life. Learn to be silent, even for a short while, so you may listen.

There is an abundance of research about one type of treatment available called ozone therapy. This is where oxygen is administered in a controlled manner into the body and, by doing so, it is possible to destroy cancers cells through oxidation whilst boosting your immune system.

This method is deemed safe to use by a trained person, but nevertheless, it is still not widely accepted by the mainstream medical profession who are deep within the pockets of drug makers and have become single-minded in their approach which, has become a desperate shame upon humanity.

This method, right now, is saving lives from long-term conventional treatment. The application of ozone can be highly beneficial against many diseases and illnesses, but you won't be given this knowledge by your doctor because it does not comply with their protocol. We have to educate ourselves.

"Ozone eliminates... viruses and bacteria from blood, human and stored... Medical ozone is successfully used on AIDS, Herpes, Hepatitis, Mononucleosis, Cirrhosis of the liver, Gangrene, Cardiovascular Disease, Arteriosclerosis, High Cholesterol, Cancerous Tumours, Lymphomas, Leukaemia... Highly effective on Rheumatoid and other Arthritis, Allergies of all types... Improves Multiple Sclerosis, ameliorates Alzheimer's Disease, Senility, and Parkinson's... Effective on Protists, Colitis, Prostrate, Candidiasis, Trichomoniasis, Cystitis; Externally, ozone is effective in treating Acne, bums, leg ulcers, open sores and wounds, Eczema, and fungus."

These results were from many different clinics and repeated year after year.

"Despite all this, the media still barrages us with sad pleas for money constantly so our medical establishment can "Find a cure" for these diseases. Well, if myself, only one man with a computer and a telephone, can find all this documentation I really don't think the medical establishment with all its money and vast resources is looking very hard. Do you?" - Ed McCabe

Chapter 9
The Incredible Healing Properties of Cannabis

This is by far the most controversial of all medications. Being the least known about medicine within the general public, it has seen a disproportionate amount of propaganda regarding its consumption recreationally or specifically for medicinal and therapeutic use within the last 100 years. Ever since campaigns launched in the 1930s by then FBI Narcotics Chief Harry Anslinger, the seed had been planted in society's mind that cannabis was evil and that it sent you insane. The promotion of "Reefer Madness" videos and Anslinger's racist obsessions for eradicating a misunderstood plant set the minds of nations against a plant that has been of great use throughout the ages. In 1928, cannabis within the UK was made illegal after signing the Geneva Convention on narcotics control in 1925. There was no lobbying either for or against its use from the public and there wasn't even a parliamentary debate on the matter. We are still at the mercy of such an unjust law today.

Cannabis is a most intriguing plant and possibly one of the greatest gifts to us from the natural world. It has been used by humans for at least 5000 years and was labelled by the Greeks as a *"panacea"*, meaning a cure-all drug. Sacred Hebrew texts refer to cannabis being used and was commonly known as kaneh-bosm. Evidence of the Hebrew use of cannabis was established in 1936 by Sulla Benet, a little-known Polish etymologist from the Institute of Anthropological Sciences in Warsaw. The word 'cannabis' was generally thought to be of Scythian origin, but Benet showed that it has a much earlier origin in Semitic languages like Hebrew, and that it appears several times throughout the Old Testament. Benet explained that, *"in the original Hebrew text of the Old Testament there are references to hemp, both as incense, which was an integral part of religious celebration, and as an intoxicant."* Benet demonstrated that the word for cannabis is kaneh Bosm, also rendered in traditional Hebrew as kane or kannada. The root kn in this construction means "reed" or "hemp", while bosm means "aromatic". This word appears five times in the Old Testament; in the books of Exodus, the Song of Songs, Isaiah, Jeremiah, and Ezekiel. The shamanistic Asher priestesses of pre-reformation Jerusalem mixed cannabis resins with those from myrrh, balsam, frankincense, and perfumes, and then anointed their skins with the mixture as well as burned it.

THEN THE LORD SAID TO MOSES, "TAKE THE FOLLOWING FINE

SPICES: 500 SHEKELS OF LIQUID MYRRH, HALF AS MUCH OF FRAGRANT CINNAMON, 250 SHEKELS OF KANNABOSM, 500 SHEKELS OF CASSIA - ALL ACCORDING TO THE SANCTUARY SHEKEL - AND A HIND OF OLIVE OIL. MAKE THESE INTO A SACRED ANNOITING OIL, A FRAGRANT BLEND, THE WORK OF A PERFUMER. [7] - EXODUS 30:22-33

Cannabis has been used by every civilisation across the globe for thousands of years. Its healing benefits and knowledge on how to cultivate such an extraordinary plant has been passed down from generation to generation. It seems strange to me that so many have benefited from cannabis use up until the prohibition of it in the early part of the last century, and that prohibition of a natural plant that grows almost anywhere on Earth is still outlawed to this day for completely incorrect and unjust reasons leaving the real truth unknown to many, especially those who strongly oppose its use.

It is becoming clear to countless people within science and medicine that cannabis prescribed correctly has incredible results with few to no side effects. Science is also backing claims through present and decade old research in understanding how this simple plant can heal so many disorders. Cannabinoids (compounds found in cannabis) have, for decades, been shown to help with chronic pain, reducing tumours, killing microbes, treating neurodegenerative disease, and helping epilepsy - all this and more from just one plant. Nearly all living species, including ourselves, have cannabinoid receptors which play a critical role in maintaining physiological functions in living organisms. Every man, woman and child has an endocannabinoid system which regulates the immune, reproductive, and nervous system by releasing cannabis-like compounds. Governments and corporations have systematically suppressed and prohibited a plant that combines with existing receptors in all Earthlings. With all the research available to us today, you could go so far as to say this plant was actually put here for us. We need not base the success of therapeutic cannabis use on anecdotal statements. The scientific proof regarding its benefits and uses is largely ignored, even though we know that cannabis is a very safe drug. Some of the biggest pharmaceutical companies today that were around in the 19th and early 20th centuries had products on the shelf of pharmacists for customers to buy with cannabis ingredients in them that were highly effective and cheap to purchase. Corporations have had the need in greed to prevent all competition that would affect profit for shareholder interests and that includes natural products, of which Mother Nature allows us, in her infinite abundance, to share with each other in this free knowledge.

Big business does not have an ethical interest in public health and they perceive natural medicine as a huge threat to their margins. You can't patent a naturally occurring plant, yet it is possible to genetically modify it and extract compounds which the companies in question can offer to the market. The plant comes in two forms; the male (hemp) produces seed which has very little psychoactive chemicals, roughly 0.005 %.

Hemp can be processed and used for a wide range of industrial purposes ranging from paper and all derivatives, fossil fuel replacement, building an entirely sustainable biodegradable home, to a well-known car manufacturer using it for their dashboards as a biodegradable plastic.

Thousands of uses for its commercial viability have been confirmed; every item made from plastic today could be made from hemp as a biodegradable and sustainably-sourced material which is as strong as steel when processed properly, and its seed is also one of the world's finest ratios of Omega-3 and 6, perfectly matching with the body's requirements for the immune system. The female plant, normally referred to as cannabis, is where the psychoactive element comes from in the form of THC (Tetrahydrocannabinol). However, cannabinoid compounds (CBDs) also present in the female plant create a synergistic effect of them both that can make a powerful cancer treatment. For a plant that has such a tainted history, its unusual safety record remains self-evident when you consider there have been no recorded deaths from human consumption! Compare this figure to alcohol and tobacco and you are left scratching your head. Please do not be fooled by the recent alleged deaths associated with smoking cannabis. The propaganda machine has used the people in the press that have tragically succumbed to death and falsely attributed cannabis as the culprit. When you look at each case closely, it is clear to see other variables involved were at play. But again, because cannabis is a controlled substance, it is used as the evil card to shape perception and further restrict its use.

"Tetrahydrocannabinol is a very safe drug. Laboratory animals (rats, mice, dogs, monkeys) can tolerate doses of up to 1,000 mg/kg

(milligrams per kilogram). This would be equivalent to a 70 kg person swallowing 70 grams of the drug -- about 5,000 times more than is required to produce a high. Despite the widespread illicit use of cannabis there are very few if any instances of people dying from an overdose. In Britain, official government statistics listed five deaths from cannabis in the period 1993-1995 but on closer examination these proved to have been deaths due to inhalation of vomit that could not be directly attributed to cannabis (House of Lords Report, 1998). By comparison with other commonly used recreational drugs these statistics are impressive." [8]

Medicinal grade cannabis is still, even today with all the medical advancements and pharmacology, one of the safest drugs in the world to use and is well-documented for being so.

Cannabis has, in studies around the globe since the 19th century, proved effective against arthritis, AIDS, asthma, glaucoma, back pain, migraine, cancer, multiple sclerosis, and many, many more ailments.

Lies spread by institutes with vested interests in petrochemicals and biotech, and certainly the paper industries alongside cotton farming, have succeeded in eradicating cannabis use in favour of producing inferior quality products. We have been prevented from expanding our knowledge and truly understanding this amazing plant because of industry leaders and the narrow minds of the past. Cannabis was very much part of mainstream medicine up until the 1930s; it was highly effective against many common ailments and easily purchased over the counter in any pharmacy. Because of the unjust laws against cannabis usage, pharmaceutical companies are producing yet evermore synthetic drugs for an organic world. A drug called Marinol, which is in capsule form, utilises only one part of the therapeutic herb that has been synthesised. The plant in its natural state has a THC value of between 2-20%; compare this with Marinol which is 98% pure and you get a very unbalanced drug. Other chemical compounds work together with THC in cannabis to counteract the negative effects but none of these compounds exist in Marinol, rendering it another unintelligent offering from the profit labs. This manufactured drug is very expensive to create, and thus a cost-prohibitive process. The procedures involved use preservatives like methylene and polypropylene whilst paramenthide (PMD), a main derivative, has caused frequent explosions in laboratories. What a huge effort to imitate that which already exists in nature. As always, a fake is no substitute for the real thing.

The big problem with Marinol is the length of time for relief to happen; as it is ingested orally, it can take up to 90 minutes and peak therapeutic effects are within 2-4 hours. Compare this to less than 5 minutes from inhaling the vapours of cannabis, whereby a user can self-regulate the strength needed and stop inhaling when peak is reached. When taking a capsule, you are at the mercy of capsule breakdown and absorption into the blood. Marinol has 4 associated deaths, has a warning about overdosing, and its use within our system of healthcare is limited to only treating chemo victims from vomiting and AIDS sufferers who cannot eat. Yet again, we are treating the symptoms and not the root source of the problem.

Sativex, a concentrated form of whole cannabis, is prescribed on the NHS, although it's very hard to get. Why? What are these offerings but a profitable substitute for nature's real deal?

"The DEA's Administrative Law Judge, Francis Young concluded: "In strict medical terms marijuana is far safer than many foods we commonly consume. For example, eating 10 raw potatoes can result in a toxic response. By comparison, it is physically impossible to eat enough marijuana to induce death. Marijuana in its natural form is one of the safest therapeutically active substances known to man. By any measure of rational analysis marijuana can be safely used within the supervised routine of medical care." [9]

"UK Home Secretary David Blunkett announced in July 2002 that "We must concentrate our efforts on the drugs that cause the most harm, while sending a credible message to young people. I will therefore ask Parliament to reclassify cannabis from Class B to Class C. I have considered the recommendations of the Home Affairs Committee, and the advice given me by the ACMD medical experts that the current classification of cannabis is disproportionate in relation to the harm that it causes." [10]

Those wishing not to inhale carcinogenic smoke from cannabis can use a clever device called a vaporiser, which heats the herb just enough to release a smokeless vapour and is then breathed in. This method is great for asthma and bronchial problems as the drug dilates your arteries, increasing blood flow, unlike smoking tobacco which restricts it. Vaporising combats any preconceptions that the drug can lead to cancer or lung disease, as the herb is heated to below the point of combustion where noxious smoke and associated toxins are produced. This drug is well-documented for halting most diseases and preventing tumour growth by attacking cancerous cells and strengthening the immune system. This is not new information that I am providing here; the US conducted studies into medical uses for cannabis back in the early seventies, but President Gerald Ford shut down all public research and granted exclusive rights for pharmaceutical companies to continue testing cannabis in an attempt to develop a synthetic version. In 1983, the Reagan Bush administration ordered the destruction of all files relating to cannabis research, including compendiums in libraries! Why destroy information regarding a natural plant if it supposedly has no purpose other than being a plant? Jack Herer's book *"The Emperor Wears No Clothes"* states that *"we know that large amounts of information have since disappeared."* [11]

Hemp, cannabis, marijuana, blow, pot, puff, weed, whatever your label of this heavenly plant - if the unjust laws were removed that bans this natural elixir, our world could be filled with less suffering, less pollution, and more profitable beneficial industries that could lead us into a new golden age of understanding and respect.

The BMA (British Medical Association) has, within the last 20 years, used the drug to treat tumours with very good results and yet, have you read any of this information on the front page of newspapers celebrating the good properties of cannabis?

Harvard University has recently - in 2011 - released results conducted on mice using the active ingredient in cannabis (THC) and they reported both a 50% plus reduction in tumour size and a halt toward cancerous growth for common lung cancer. Aggressive lung cancers are resistant to chemotherapy but not, it seems, for a natural plant you could grow in your back garden. Understanding the implications of humans *"legally"* growing a plant in their own garden to cure cancer in less than 12 months with no surgery, chemo, radiotherapy, or steroids is truly mind-blowing.

I would really like the reader to contemplate what effects this would have on the cancer drug industry as a whole if this could be achieved in a free world. We would never need to use the taxpayer's money again, fighting a war that can already be won. It's happening right now; with our money being wasted funding medical fraud whilst the suffering of many continues. It does not have to be this way, as the use of Cannabis matched with the correct diet can kill cancer cells safely.

As of early 2012, cannabis is still classed as Schedule 1 - a drug with no medical value - under the 1971 Misuse of Drugs Act. What I find interesting is the behaviour of society toward cannabis and its legal alternative, alcohol. We demonise cannabis use and yet at the same time celebrate the intoxication of alcohol. We lead by example apparently and yet adults slosh back volumes of alcohol at parties, barbecues, and most daytime events in full view of children. This is oddly accepted within society, even though we know that alcohol abuse is right at the top of the damaging drugs list. I find this utterly contradictory when drinkers condemn cannabis smokers. Being an ex-smoker myself for over 20 years, I can honestly say, from my own personal observations, that I have seen more devastation to the mind, soul, and body from social drinking events in 1 night than 2 decades within the cannabis smoking cultures around the world. We have been gravely misled, and my opinion is that our perceptions are not always our own. A hard-driven agenda coming from a failed war on drugs has shaped many minds in society and helped to demonise that which could prove helpful.

Cannabis oil

Rick Simpson is a Canadian hailed as the bringer and re-discoverer of therapeutic oil to great public attention. His story should be far more publicised than it has been to date and the results he has witnessed with others, along with his continued efforts, are certainly nothing short of extraordinary. He is currently in exile from his own country of Canada because the authorities want to charge him with growing and supplying cannabis, albeit purely for medicinal therapeutic benefit, which he didn't make a single penny from for offering his medicine to his fellow citizens. He approached health and government officials regarding the benefits of cannabis oils asking for recognition of an amazing plant, only to be silenced by the establishment. He is unwillingly somewhere in Europe now, acting as a cannabis campaigner. Further insight and updates into Rick and his knowledge can be found on the internet. Rick's case is by no means an isolated example of people benefitting from the medicinal qualities of cannabis and, since his testimony to the world, thousands of people have benefitted from this elixir. There is an abundance of research that proves the amazing medicinal benefits of cannabis, and there are more than enough studies in existence that would ,if the plant were not illegal, pass government and health regulations to be used by the public as a therapeutic and safe drug. To step beyond our current knowledge is difficult when entering new unfamiliar territory as our fear takes over too much of the time and we forget how intelligent we really are. There are so many distractions in our lives today that it seems inconceivable at times to dedicate our efforts in truly understanding the world we live in and share this knowledge with each other. In my opinion, we have been manipulated into this slumber by governing entities using every possible tactic at certainly the highest levels of authority to render us helpless, but we are not.

"You can fool some of the people all of the time, and all of the people some of the time, but you cannot fool all of the people all of the time." - Abraham Lincoln

Chapter 10
Conclusion

As, hopefully, you may be aware by now, there are great lengths at which information is suppressed and misinterpreted. Propaganda plays a dark hand in shaping how we react to the deviation of mainstream thinking. You may be wondering to yourself by now why, if this knowledge is true, I have never heard of its many uses and why it is not being used in hospitals all over the land. The answer to this is that which makes the world go round; money, and ultimately power through the obliteration of all natural competition. Many people are unaware of these events happening all around them. I, too, having no prior knowledge of medicine, fully believed that doctors had every resource in their power to make my family well when illness arrives and that no conflict of interests between patient and drug manufacturers existed. We are guinea pigs to the pharmaceutical industry, a business that fails to recognise the importance of natural cures and has absolute disregard to the existing quantity outside of patient protection. Society's perception that cancer is still incurable has stemmed from the belief in a myth, and it is this distorted view that gives energy to the machine of industry that will not stop unless we change our perception of thought. Restrictions currently in place limits the methods a doctor may use to teach and treat a patient.

There are grey areas in long-term treatment that are operating on a level which causes far more suffering than eradicating disease and infection. The arrogance of man to exclude from healing all mediums which should be exploited is devastating to our survival. This orchestrated system in censorship of information has been in place for a long time. The authorities in place to protect us have assisted in the prevention of so many effective treatment protocols, extending their power to discredit, threaten, ridicule and revoke licenses. So impressive the campaign of silence has become that the general public are tragically cut off from remarkable and dedicated professionals showing us there are other ways to treat and heal. As a society, we have embraced the large corporations involved in setting their very own parameters of safety, and we are, in effect, conditioned to believe we are receiving the most beneficial methods of healing the body needs when at dis-ease. Licences of genuine doctors, physicians, and healers who had created pioneering alternative medical work in the fight against cancer lost out, appallingly so, and so has humanity.

The painful part is that the great work achieved often gets buried and is so rarely considered in teaching. Ending disease is not in the interests of those involved with pharmaceuticals and chronic disease management. By creating the term "quackery" in the early 20th century, it was easy to label everything that was not Big Pharma a mere fraud and, although there was then and still are many health frauds in the world, the seed in people's minds had been sown for the truth to become blurred. The foundations were laid then for the masses to believe all that corporations had to say, as they had government backing and the biased statistics to fool most of society. The true "quackery" is what happens to be the acceptable and current medications we consume collectively today with little question to its true benefits.

The network that is in place now for the treatment of serious illness is staggeringly flawed, but it does not take long to educate ourselves about any matter on our planet. It is only because we have been given the wrong information that we are suffering so greatly. We can change this. Big Pharma is built on the fraudulent lies that secure the wealth of the few against the ill and unwell. They exist based upon their untruths, for we have allowed them to and they have been successful at it. Our bodies were never designed to accept synthetic drugs, as we are as organic as the trees, plants, and animals in our world. Many alternative methods for treating disease in the last 100 years have been outlawed by pharmaceutical companies that are deeply entrenched in policy making within governance; not because they are unsafe, or have terrible side effects, or because little is known about each method, or protecting public safety - simply because they all threaten the global industry of symptom-masking medicine which, as we will come to understand, is perpetuating our health problems. The elimination of ALL competition is the power and success behind any corporate entity operating for profit on behalf of its shareholders.

Our psychological mind-set has been unknowingly manipulated to explicitly render our own power as human masters of own bodies obsolete. We are getting sicker for longer because we are losing control of our own intelligence and the confidence and ability to help enable change within our own lives. This can change like the flick of a light switch, providing we are allowed to investigate without prohibition the possibilities attainable here on Earth.

Our health care system's long road is full of potholes that do not show any signs of healing just yet, and the privatisation of healthcare within the UK will see an explosion of expensive medication that will fail the rich as it does now while excluding the poor. Bureaucracy, treachery, greed, and control loiter in the minds of Big Business, and that is what the health system has become. In my opinion, controlling families such as the Rockefellers and Rothschilds have had a powerful dominating role in suppressing what could be common knowledge and advantageous for a mature developed world and these elite families and their monetary ties have prevented truths from reaching lower classes and society in general. Hollywood's dramatisations of psychotics and what they look like are a false illusion within society; however, our world is run by psychopaths of industry. The real psychopaths are the leading figures of power seldom seen who have little or no empathy or compassion for humanity. Political parties create more legislation and master misinformation for citizens to divulge and manufacture consent to. Governments are reading the scripts set out by the ringmasters who are above governance with zero accountability. As long as these powerful organisations exist, so will subtle tyranny toward those who wish to get well and be free to choose how they get well. We are continually basing our healthcare on erroneous statistics and government targets that are inadequate and, considering the scale of our health issues, this has lead the health services to develop insistent pen-pushing and further drastic cutbacks that prevent real healthcare from being administered in far more cost-effective fashion. We cannot even keep our hospitals clean today. The practical action required to problem solve is quickly being dissolved from all rungs of the working ladder. By destroying knowledge and pushing out common sense, the system can rely on the fear and scripted guidance of its sleepy servants.

The modification of humans has created new symptoms with labels that most share common detriments in toxic overload, inflammation, and dietary deficiency. Alternative medicines are not the alternative at all; natural medicine healing has been around since the dawn of mankind. Its use in human history has been very much the normal way of treating health problems to great effect within all cultures globally, historically, and presently. Many of the effective ways of treating outside of orthodox medicine are becoming lost to the people, and is becoming widely visible by the lack of practical knowhow in new generations that are not being taught how to look after their health. The greater reliance on convenient packaged modern medicine has quickly become a commercial enterprise which is open for abuse, leading to addiction from prescription drugs with their identifiable and increasing side effects and to the continued reliance upon synthetic pills which advocates proclaim to halt the ageing process, cure disease, or save us from both. They are junk.

There is an empowering responsibility associated with simply knowing. Sometimes, simple human observation can account for a lot and we should not discount it from existing policies. We are individually personally responsible for the treatment of our bodies while we are alive and able, and the simple actions we can commit to against illness have been shown to determine whether we prosper in health or not.

In the last century a huge leap in medical technology and scientific research appears to have furthered our understanding of the human form, though there is much still to re-discover about the unique ways of healing that are ignored by organisations as they challenge the status quo.

A strong grip of corporate interests in the field of medicine exists and the existence of shareholders has a major influence in which drug should be favoured and adhered to for society's woes.

It is up to you, the reader, to determine for yourself what the truth is and can be, no other being can tell you the truth or define it, as we have to see it for ourselves. The writer is not pushing a belief, or implying any evidence found here is the only way of resolve. Science, by its very nature, is ever-evolving and correcting once held truths or untruths. Solutions can become lost in the ether of time when correct science is prevented by biased attitudes of servitude. We have been cultured to believe that expert scientific proof is the governing body of all truths, but who are the experts?

Science is as much manipulated for profit growth as is the current private banking system. We have given up our critical thought and the ability to question, at length, the nature of precise outcomes from mainstream views at our loss. We have also become apathetic and helped to enforce the belief that an expert somewhere on a payroll is far more intelligent than we could ever be. We can take responsibility for ourselves.

If anything, the writer simply wants to demonstrate the idea of something different from that which we have come to accept as acceptable. We should employ excellence from sustainable resources in a manner that does not accept the average, but strives and thrives to better our health and environment for all of humanity. We are an indoctrinated and tamed society that is often fooled in our youth, taking with us into adulthood the beating drum of misinformation and illusions we believe we cannot solve. We can.

Taking back our responsibility is key and we must remember that we really are human beings and not just testing mediums for corporate entities. Amnesia is rife in today's nations; however, we are finally remembering that, by using nature with its inherent qualities and safety, alongside science and technology, we will unlock the answers for all beings here in this world.

Written and compiled by a human being living on Earth.

References:

[1] 2001 The Soil Association and sustain: The alliance for better food and farming
non-sustaining

[2] Nenah Sylver "The Rife Handbook"

[3] Health Protection Agency, Notifications and deaths in England and Wales, 1940-2008

[4] Luby, Stephen P., Sabina Wall-to-wall, Daniel R. Feint, John Painter, Ward Biller, Harsh Altai, and Robert M. Orchestra."Effect of Hand washing on Child Health: A Randomised Controlled Trial." The Lancet 366, no. 9481 (July 16, 2005): 225–233. soi:10.1016/S0140-6736(05)66912-7.

[5] Relative trends in hospitalizations and mortality among infants by the number of vaccine doses and age, based on the Vaccine Adverse Event Reporting System (VAERS), 1990-2010. Hum Exp Toxicology October 2012; 31(10): 1012-1021.

[6] Chemotherapy study published 6th August 2012 in " Nature Medicine"

[7] The books of Exodus, the Song of Songs, Isaiah, Jeremiah, and Ezekiel.

[8] P46-Inverse, Leslie L., PhD, FRS, "The Science of Marijuana" (London, England: Oxford University Press, 2000), p. 178, citing House of Lords, Select Committee on Science and Technology, "Cannabis -- The Scientific and Medical Evidence" (London, England: The Stationery Office, Parliament, 1998).

[9] P47- US Department of Justice, Drug Enforcement Agency, "In the Matter of Marijuana Rescheduling Petition," [Docket #86-22], (September 6, 1988), p. 57.

[10] P47-"'All Controlled Drugs Harmful, All Will Remain Illegal' - Home Secretary," News Release, Office of the Home Secretary, Government of the United Kingdom, July 10, 2002, from the web at http://213.219.10.30/n_storyboard?item_id=143 last accessed July 31, 2002.

[11] "The emperor wears no clothes" Jack Herer

Recommended Reading:

Jason Vale "The Juice Master's Ultimate Fast Food"
This book can show you that which no pill can ever do for your health.

Ty Bollinger "Step Outside the Box"

Professor Jane Plant "Your Life In Your Hands"

Philip Day "Cancer: Why We're Still Dying to Know the Truth"

Ed McCabe "Flood Your Body with Oxygen"

Charlotte Gerson "The Gerson Therapy"

Valerie Ann Wormwood "The Fragrant Pharmacy"
This book is exceptionally useful for using essential oils, and I use it every week for its simple yet effective knowledge.

Christina England "Shaken Baby Syndrome Or Vaccine Induced Encephalitis"

Dr Richard Halvorsen "The Truth About Vaccines: Making the Right Decision for Your Child"

Suzanne Humphries MD and Roman Bystrianyk "Dissolving Illusions: Disease, Vaccines, and The Forgotten History"

"Living Energies: Viktor Schauberger's Brilliant Work with Natural Energy Explained" by Callum Coats (1 Sep 2001)

Jack Herer "The Emperor Wears No Clothes"

Catherine J. Frompovich "A Cancer Answer: Holistic Breast Cancer Management, A Guide to Effective & Non-Toxic Treatments"

"The Essential Herbs Handbook" Lesley Bremness

"The New Holistic Herbal" David Hoffman

"Calling of an Angel" Gary L. Glum

"Rick Simpson Oil - Nature's Answer for Cancer" Rick Simpson

Nenah Sylver "The Rife Handbook"

Documentaries:

"The Beautiful Truth"

"Healing Cancer From Inside Out"

"Cancer - The Forbidden Cures"

"Ride with Larry"

"Run From The Cure"

"World without Cancer"

"The Truth About Cancer"

"The Gerson Therapy - Charlotte Gerson on Curing Cancer"

"Shattering Cancer with Resonant Frequencies"

"Genetic Roulette"

"Seeds of Death"

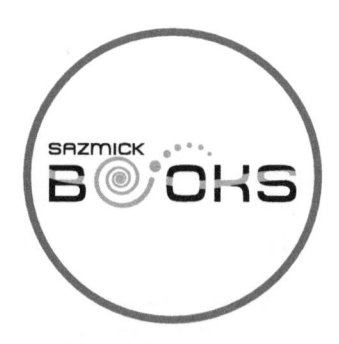

Self-Publishing Your Book Made Easy!

Sazmick Books offer self-publishing and marketing services to authors of most genres. We help to fulfill your ambition of getting your work from typed or written manuscript, into a printed book or E-book with customisable add-ons.

Simple packages, Stunning books.

Chat with us and get your book on the road today!

www.sazmickbooks.com

For All Your Self-Publishing Needs